LIMITED OR LAZY
LIMITED OR LAZY
LIMITED OR LAZY

A cookbook for all

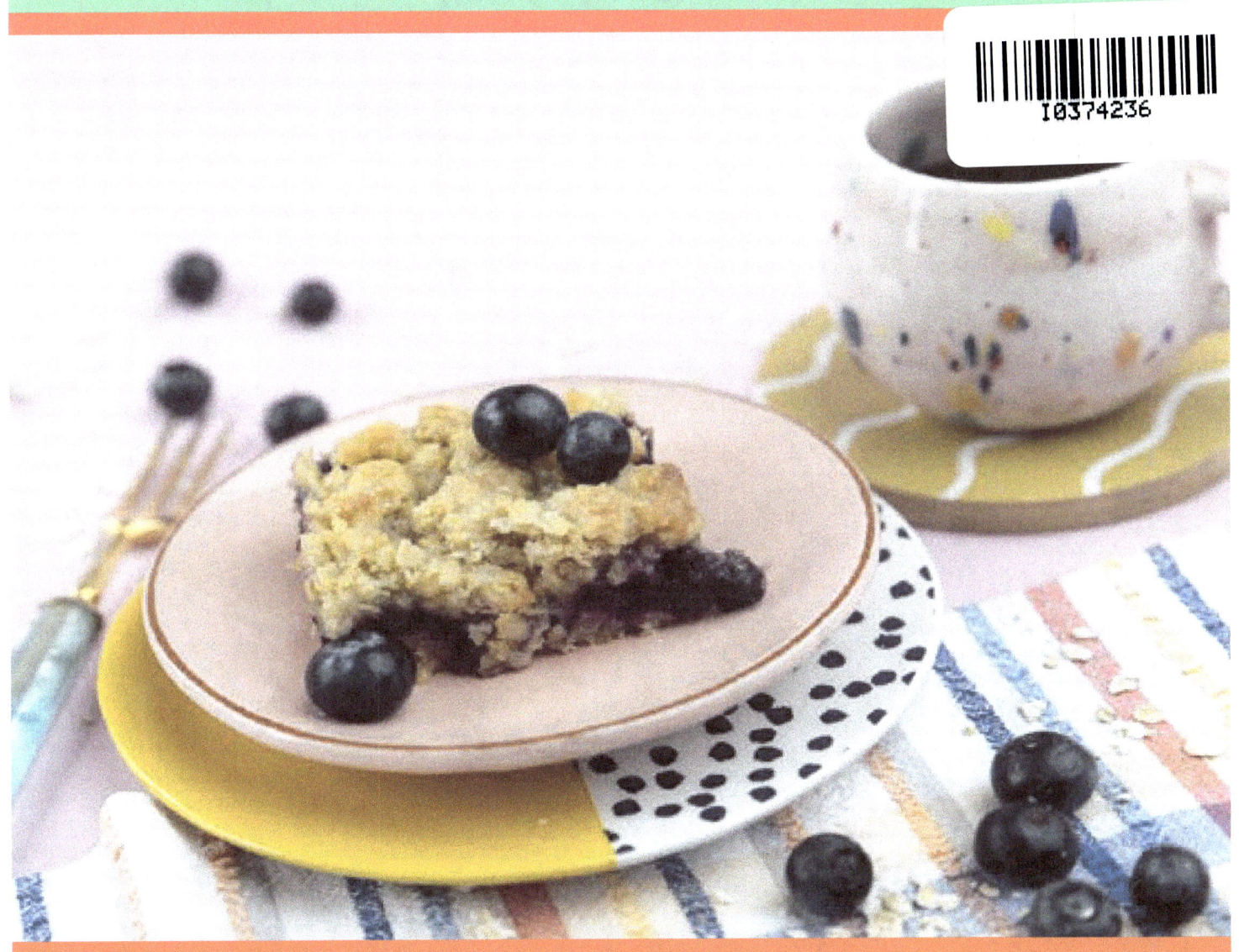

By Lynn Smith

Illustrated by Catherine Christie

LIMITED OR LAZY
LIMITED OR LAZY
LIMITED OR LAZY

A cookbook for all

By Lynn Smith
Illustrated by Catherine Christie
Photos By David Lozowy

©2023. Lynn Smith, Catherine Christie, & David Lozowy.
All contents and artwork rights reserved.

Contents:

Kitchen Journal

Starters

Soup

Mains

Pasta

Desserts

Sweet Treats

INTRODUCTION

Are you limited, lacking in confidence or simply a little bit lazy?

Granny Smith has come up with some top tips and recipes to help you shine in the kitchen.

A recipe book like no other is how I perceive it.

Having been struck down with Multiple Sclerosis 7 years ago I had to give up the job I loved as the head of a Home Economics department as I was unable to cope with the pace and practical element of the subject. My thoughts as a result of this was to turn my hand (the one that was working properly, haha) into producing a recipe book to help people who love cooking but struggle for some reason to carry out all the tasks from scratch. It is with this in mind my insight came into using pre-prepared ingredients and labour saving equipment to help produce the home cooked meals I've always loved to make for myself and my family.

Having worked for over 30 years teaching kids to cook I decided it was time to turn my experiences into helping others to become more independent and productive in the kitchen whilst achieving their goals in making spectacular food.

Having developed a training kitchen and restaurant and run many fundraising Gala Dinners whilst in post my enthusiasm for helping people achieve their optimum and boost their confidence was evident.

This book not only caters for people like me who are a bit limited physically but it is also intended for those of you who lack time in the kitchen but still want to impress. It's great for people who are very busy with for example a young family, work commitments and so on, the list is endless. It's also a really good book for students who may be lacking in experience and learning how to make ends meet on a limited budget.

An added bonus is that it is also a good recipe book if you're just having one of those lazy days but still want to impress hence the title.

The Kitchen Journal section within the book also gives you some of my top tips to help you achieve your goal.

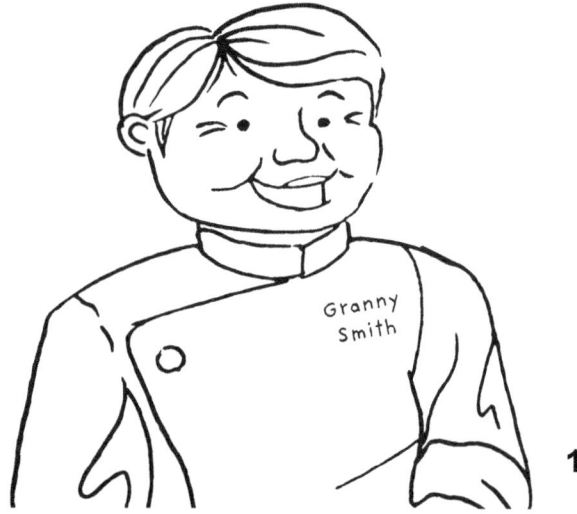

The Kitchen Journal

The following kitchen journal will help you out with what ingredients would be useful to have in your cupboards as well as giving you some top tips to help you succeed and impress in the kitchen.

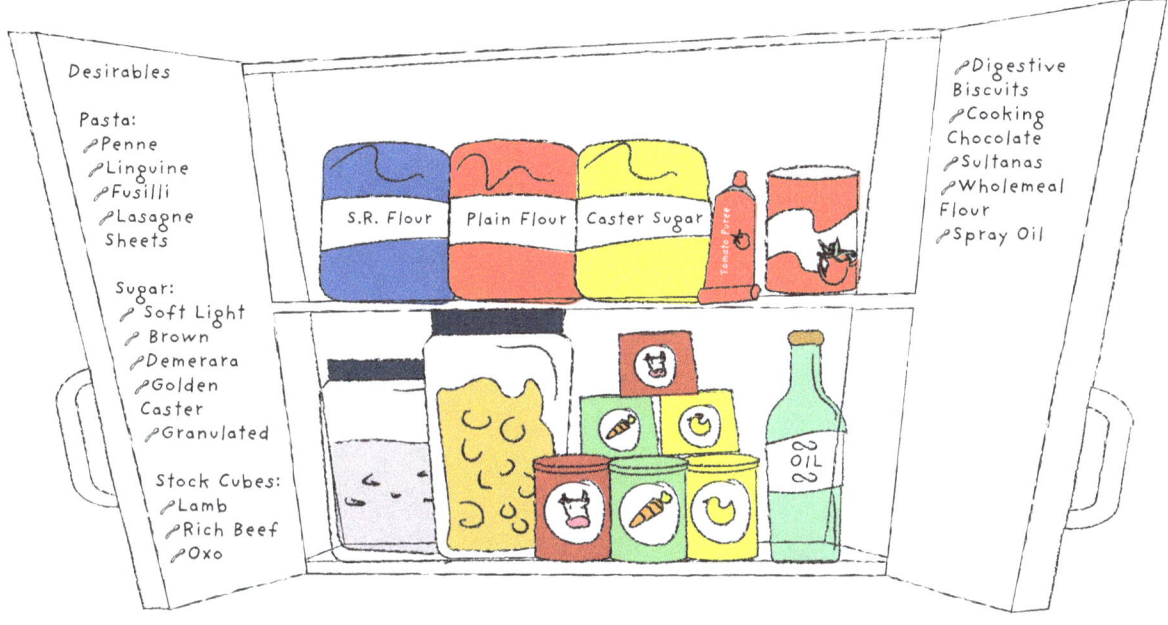

Essentials

Top shelf

Self-Raising Flour
Plain Flour
Caster Sugar
Tomato Puree
Tinned Chopped Tomatoes

Bottom shelf

Pasta – Macaroni, Spaghetti
Rice – Long Grain or Basmati
Stock Pots or Cubes –
- Chicken
- Beef
- Vegetable

Gravy Granules –
- Beef
- Chicken
- Vegetable

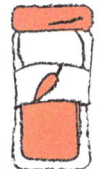 Chilli Powder   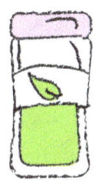 Mixed Herbs   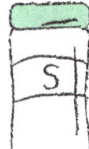 Salt   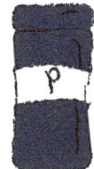 Pepper

FRIDGE INGREDIENTS:

Essential:

Margarine

Milk

Cheese (grated)

Desirable:

Cheese — Cream Cheese, Mozzarella

Butter (slightly salted)

FREEZER INGREDIENTS:

Essential:

Pre - diced Onion

Desirable:

Pre - sliced Peppers

Pre - diced Garlic

Pre - diced Chilli

Pre - chopped Basil instead of fresh or frozen

Pre - chopped Coriander)

Pre - sliced Mushrooms

NB: You can use jars or tubes of Garlic, Chilli, Basil and Coriander.

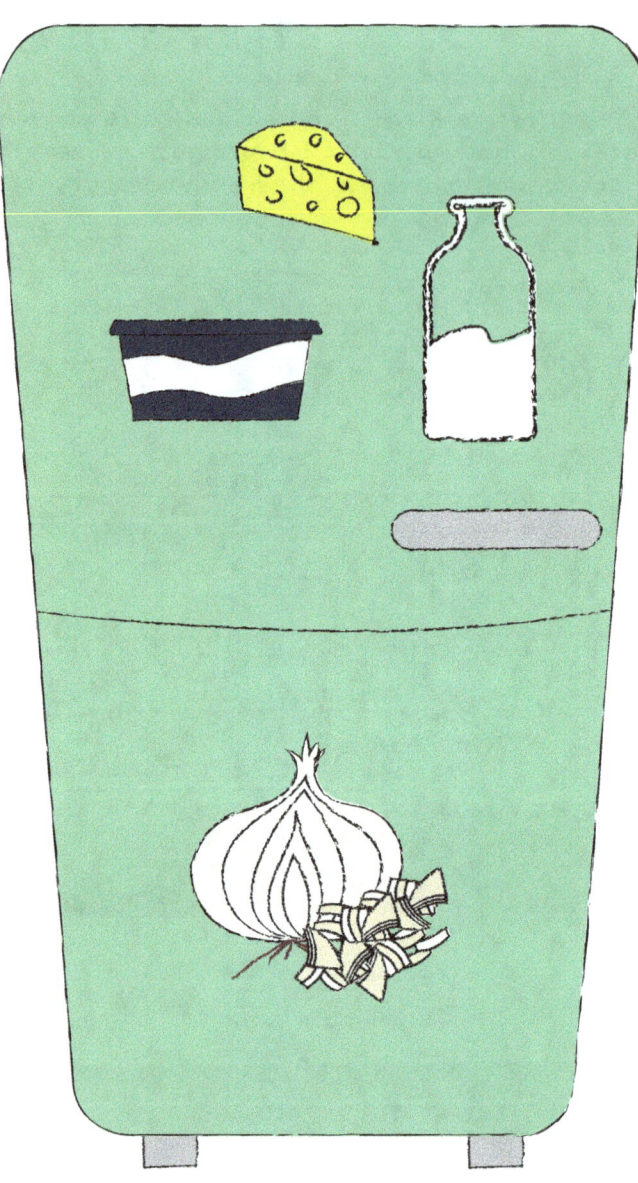

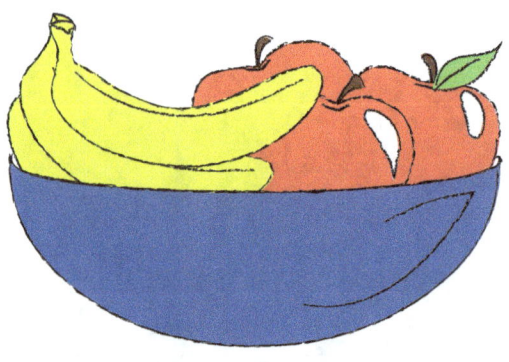

FRUIT BOWL:

Desirable:

Bananas

Apples

Ingredients preferred for some of the recipes:

Strong Flour

Cornflour

Dark Brown Sugar

Get Yourself Equipped

Equipment:

Essential:

Scales

Cup (holds 175mls liquid)

Mug (holds 250mls liquid)

Tablespoon

Dessertspoon

Teaspoon

Woodenspoon

Large Bowl

Small Bowl

Sieve

Plate

Measuring Jug

Vegetable Knife

Vegetable Peeler

Baking Tray / Swiss Roll Tin

Round Sandwich Tin (15cm)

Cooling Tray

Tin Foil

Greaseproof paper

Clingfilm

Desirable:

Electric Hand Mixer

Food Processor

Spatula

Palette Knife

Fish Slice

Cook's Knife (large sharp knife)

Tongs

Rolling Pin

Patty/Bun tin

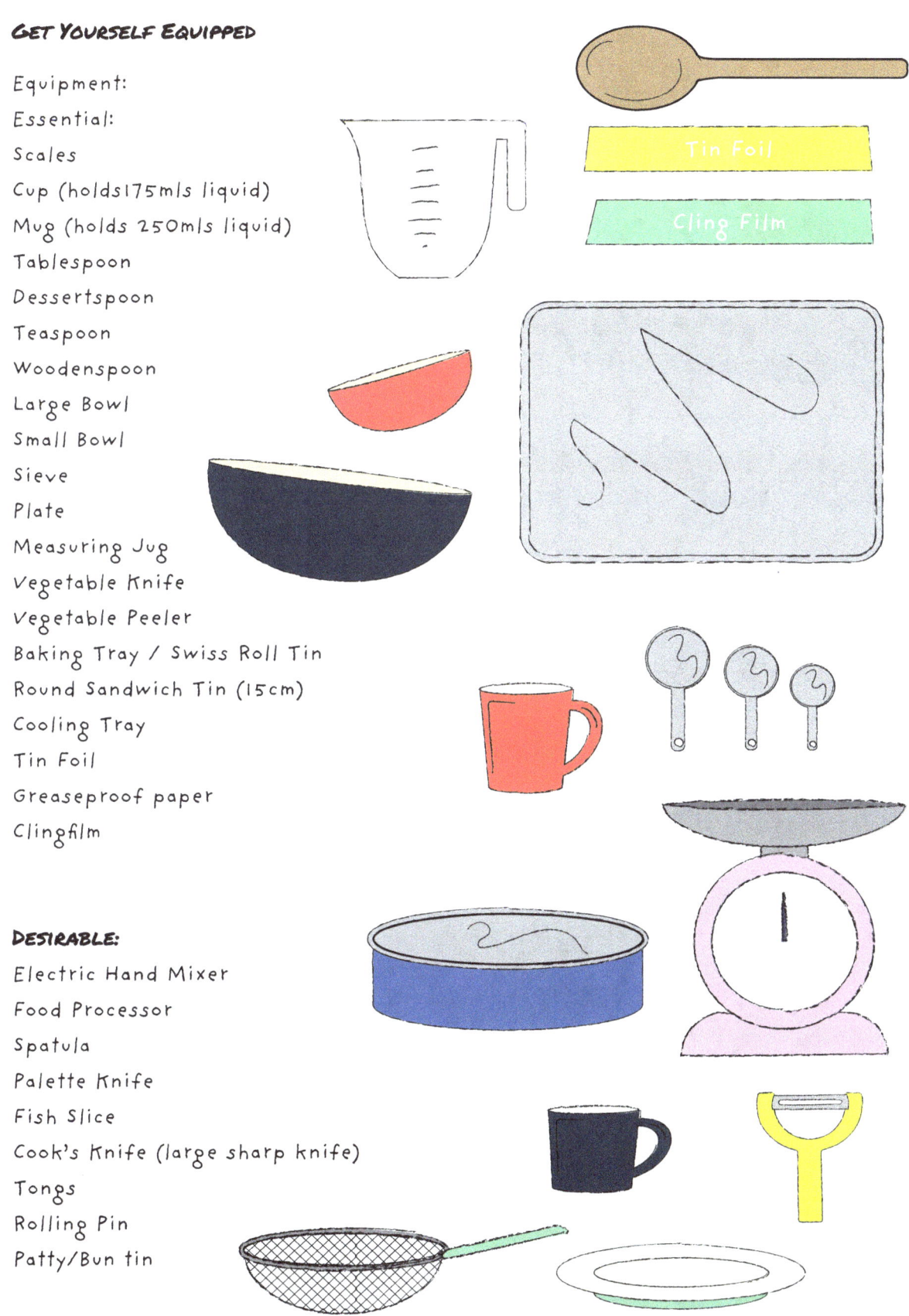

Wee Kitchen Dilemmas

Have you ever thought what to use as an alternative piece of equipment or technique?

Use the side of a flat sided wine bottle as a rolling pin. (Use a screw top bottle and have a sneaky glass of vino whilst cooking).

Instead of making a cheese/white sauce use a can of condensed soup with half a can of milk.

Place a damp net cloth or paper towel under the chopping board to prevent it moving while preparing vegetables.

Use disposable tin foil trays instead of baking trays to save the washing up.

Make your own garlic butter by mixing 50g of softened slightly salted butter with ¼ teaspoon of garlic puree / garlic granules.

Use a cup that holds 150mls of liquid and a mug that holds 250mls of liquid.

Use UHT double cream instead of fresh double cream as it won't over whip and go to butter.

Buy greaseproof loaf/cake tin liners

Use a potato masher if you have not got a hand blender or liquidise

Wash unpolished rice through a sieve to remove the starch before cooking.

Get a hold of an old fashioned tablespoon for handy measures:

1 rounded tablespoon of flour = 25g
1 slightly rounded tablespoon of sugar = 25g

(remember sugar weighs heavier than flour that's why it is slightly rounded)

KNOCK

To test if bread is ready, tap the base of it and make sure it sounds hollow.

KNOCK

Allergens - Be safe

The following allergens must now be given by law on food labels which also applies to additives, processing aids and any other substances which are present in a product.

It is important the cook recognises and makes known to the person eating their food of any allergens contained in the recipes they have made.

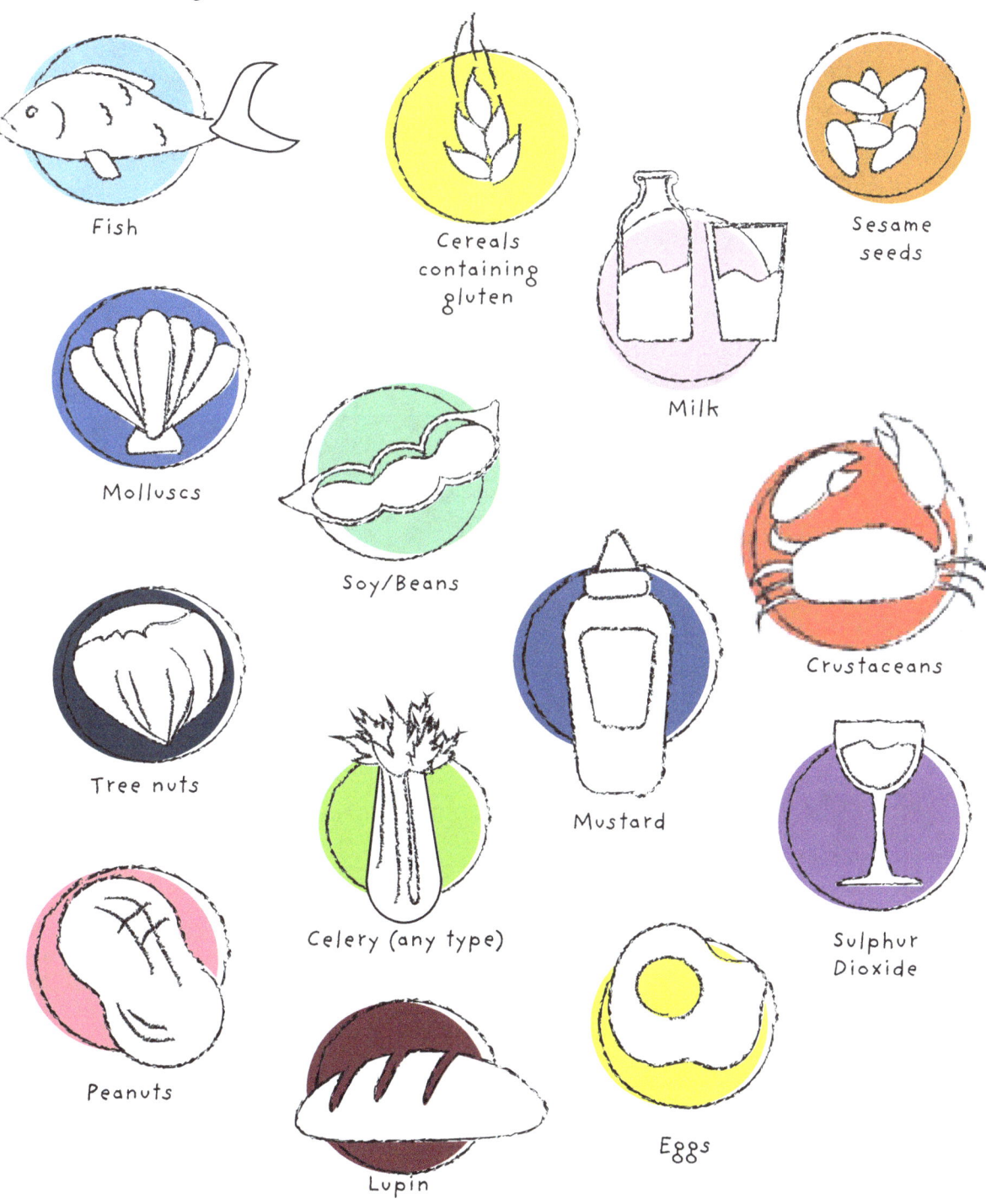

Get Those Temperatures Right

Temperature Conversion Chart

°Celsius	Gas Mark	Description
110	1/4	Very cool/ very slow
130	1/2	--
140	1	Cool
150	2	--
170	3	Very moderate
180	4	Moderate
190	5	---
200	6	Moderately hot
220	7	Hot
230	8	---
240	9	Very hot

The above temperatures are a guide, take the time to learn your oven's temperature. Every oven is different, so if in doubt go with your gut.

Microwave Oven

Know the Power Level of your microwave.

The Higher the Wattage, the quicker it cooks.

Remember to allow Standing Time (time it is still cooking whilst sitting).

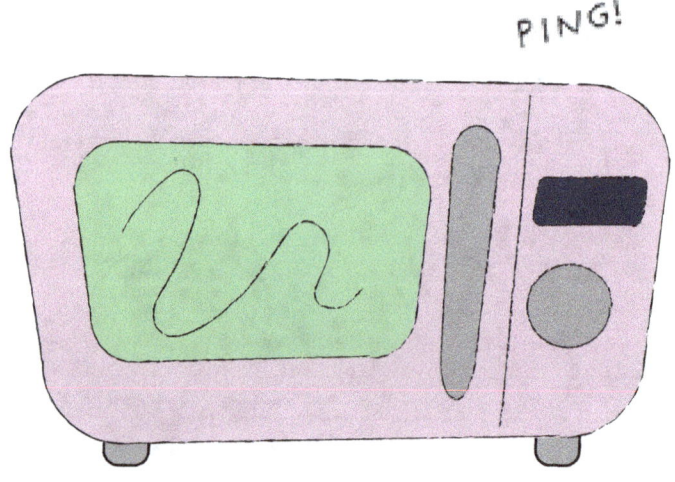

PING!

Weighing and measuring:

Handy Measures — getting it right for powder ingredients such as flour (Remember sugar weighs heavier than flour so a slightly rounded tablespoon will give 25g).

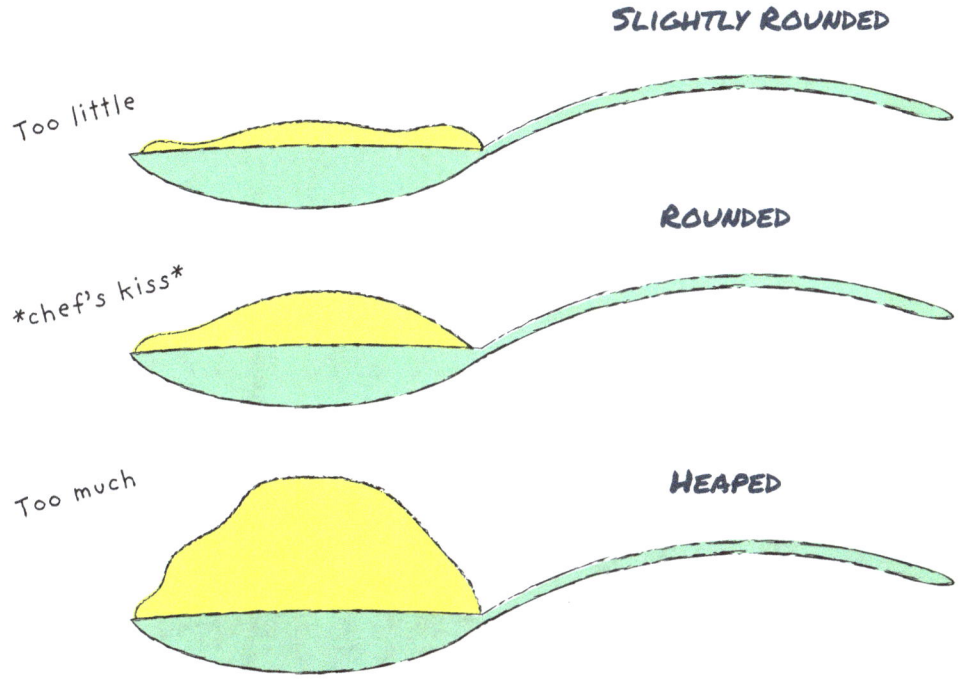

Know your Spoons

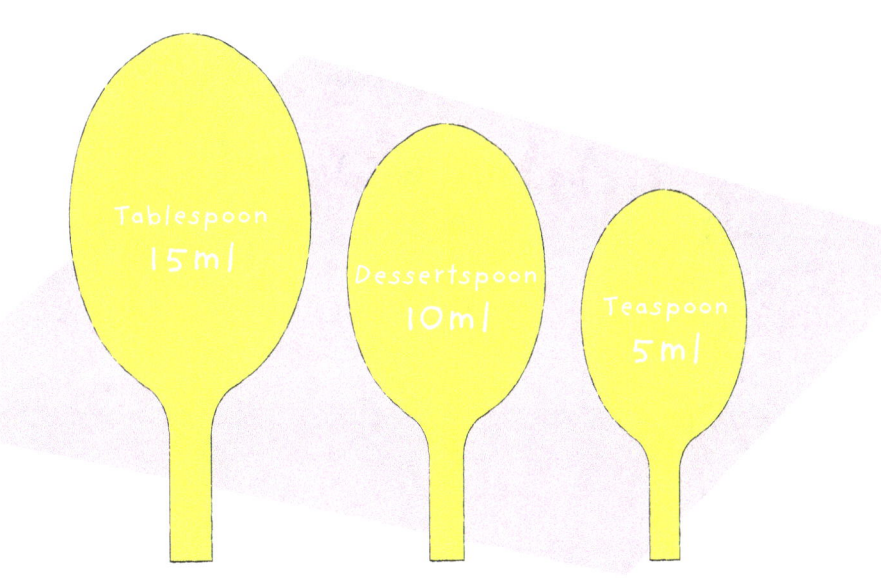

Never a problem, only a solution

Sometimes things don't work out as you planned in the kitchen. The following chapter will help you find the solution to many common kitchen errors.

The first thing to remember is...

Rule #1 Don't panic

Rule #2 Look for a solution

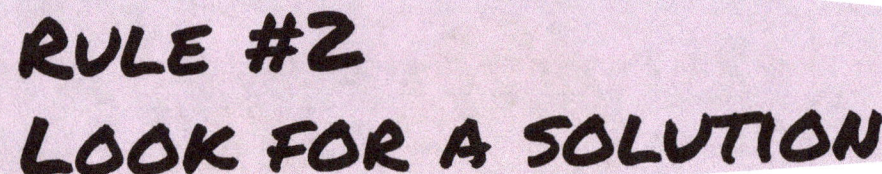

I HAVE FOUND THE SACRED TEXTS!

The cake mixture is starting to curdle

- Beat in a little of the sieved flour to stop it curdling.

Cake sinks in the middle

- During baking: Don't open oven too early.

- After it has been removed from the oven – disguise the dip in the middle by decorating it carefully.

Top of cake not browning quickly enough

- Have patience – allow it to bake at the temperature set.

- Turn the oven up slightly if you know it is cooked through and you only need it to brown otherwise you could end up with a brown crust and a raw sponge inside.

Cake sticks to inside of tin

- Before turning into the tin make sure it is greased and lined properly.

- Follow the baking time on the recipe.

- Run a knife around the inside edge of the tin to release it but make sure you don't rip the edge of the cake.

Top of cake browning too quickly, sponge not cooked

- Turn the oven down.

The fatless sponge has not risen well

Before baking make sure you:

- Weigh ingredients correctly.

- Whisk the eggs and sugar until they leave a trail on the surface.

Hint — you should be able to either draw a figure 8 or your initials on the top and it will stay there.

- Do not over fold or whisk in the flour.

After it has been baked:

- Decorate it to disguise it or start again...or use it in a trifle.

Meringues

Egg white is over whipped and starting to separate

- Throw it out and start again as the mixture will not hold its shape when piped.

Egg whites won't whisk up

Before starting make sure:
- There is no egg yolk in the bowl.
- The bowl is clean and dry.

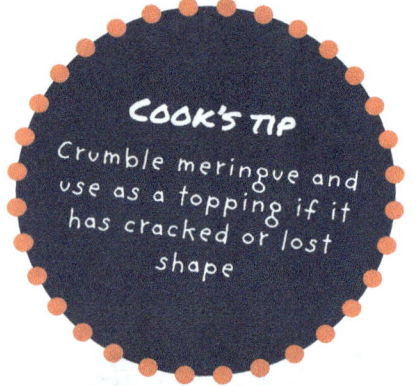

Cook's tip
Crumble meringue and use as a topping if it has cracked or lost shape

Whisked egg white is losing its shape

- Always add the sugar gradually and don't over fold it in.

Browning of dishes

Grated cheese/crumb toppings not browning quickly enough

- Place under a hot grill to brown or turn the oven up.

Dishes browning at one side

- Turn the item round in the oven so that the other side browns.

Grated cheese/crumb toppings browning too quickly

- If the dish is in the oven, loosely cover the top of it with tin foil.

(NB: Cheese will stick to the tin foil.)

Stop a dish browning too quickly

- Turn the oven/grill down.

Pasta / Rice

Rice turning sticky

Before cooking:

- Place rice in a sieve and rinse thoroughly with cold water to remove the starch.

After cooking:

- Pour into a sieve and rinse with boiling water.

Pasta over cooking

- Pour into a sieve, rinse with boiling water then stir in a little olive oil.

Rissotto sticking to the pan before rice is cooked

- Stir in a little more liquid (stock/water) and allow to reduce before serving.

Cook's Tip

Pasta should be served 'Al dente'

"Al dente" is a term used to describe pasta that's fully cooked, but not overly soft. The phrase is Italian for "to the tooth," or "to the bite" which comes from testing the pasta's consistency with your teeth.

Using the Hob

Fat in pan on fire Do not move the pan.

- Turn off the heat and cover with a fire blanket or a baking tray to exclude the air.

- Leave to cool before moving.

- DO NOT PUT WATER ON AN OIL FIRE!

Melted fat sparking or beginning to smoke

- Remove from the heat eg Slide carefully onto an unused area of the hob and allow to cool slightly before using.

- Do not add any water into the pan.

- Make sure food to be cooked is as dry as possible eg. vegetables / meat.

Sauteeing (e.g. onions / mushrooms, peppers)

- If it starts to overheat, take off heat, add a splash of COLD oil to cool the pan and stir to prevent bits burning.

- Take care not to burn garlic as it will go bitter and spoil the dish. Make sure temperature isn't too high.

PASTRY MAKING

PASTRY OVER-RUBBED IN AND GREASY

- Throw it out and start again.

Hint: if your hands are too hot, cool them by running your wrists under cold water — this will cool the blood flowing into your hands/fingers.

After cooking:

Pour into a sieve and rinse with boiling water.

PASTRY DOUGH TOO HARD TO ROLL

- Bring back to room temp if it has been in a fridge.

SHRINKAGE

- Make sure you push pastry down into the corners to stop it shrinking back too much.
- Allow to rest before trimming.

FLAN RING LINED WITH PASTRY HAS A CRACK OR HOLE IN IT OR THE SIDES ARE TOO SHORT

- Before baking:

Dampen the pastry (with water) round the hole or on the sides and seal with a piece of pastry. Flatten into shape.

- After baking:

If there is a hole in the pastry after baking, plug with a little left-over pastry (only if the hole is not too big and the flan case is to be cooked further.

- Small cracks — brush with a little egg to seal it.
- Keep any left-over pastry in the fridge to use for repairs.

WHIPPING CREAM

OVER WHIPPED AND ABOUT TO SEPARATE

- Stir in a little more cold cream or whole milk if it is just starting to go beyond piping consistency — do not beat the mixture.
- Throw it out and start again if it has started to turn to butter.

Sauces, Stews, and Soups

My sauce/stew/soup is too thick

- Add a little more liquid such as water, stock, or milk.

My sauce/stew/soup is too salty

- Add a whole peeled potato to soup to absorb the salt and remove before serving.
- Add some more liquid.

Hint – You may need to thicken it with a little cornflour blended in cold water to achieve the correct consistency.

My sauce has gone lumpy

- Beat with a whisk of hand blender.
- Sieve the sauce.
- Blend then pass through a fine sieve.
- Start again if too lumpy.

My cheese sauce has started to separate

- When making a cheese sauce, bring the sauce to the boil first then **take the pan off the heat** before adding the cheese – this will stop the cheese from separating.

(There will be enough heat in the sauce to melt the cheese).

My sauce/stew/soup is too thin

- Simmer it with the lid off until you get the correct consistency.
- Thicken with the appropriate thickening agent (eg. Cornflour, arrowroot). Blend it with a little cold water first then stirring all the time add to the soup/stew/sauce.
- Add a grated potato to soup and simmer until thickened.
- Use gravy granules – remember they can add salt.

Cook's tip

Never bring a sauce to the boil too quickly — you must have patience and allow it to come to the boil slowly and you must stir it all the time.

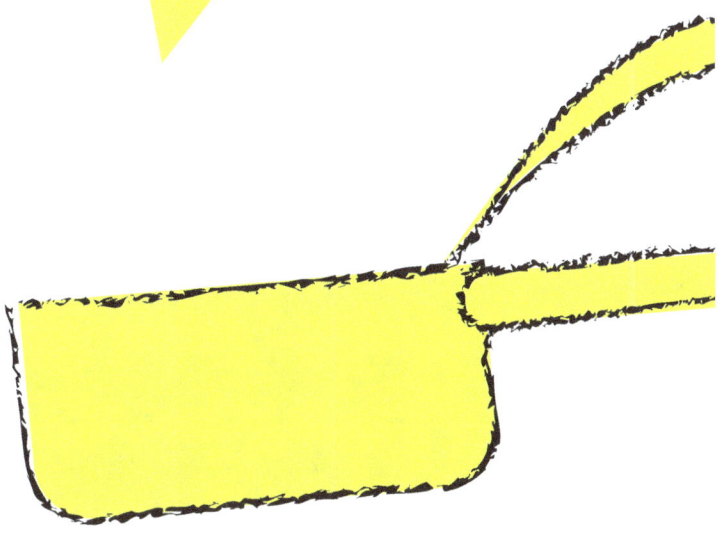

STARTERS

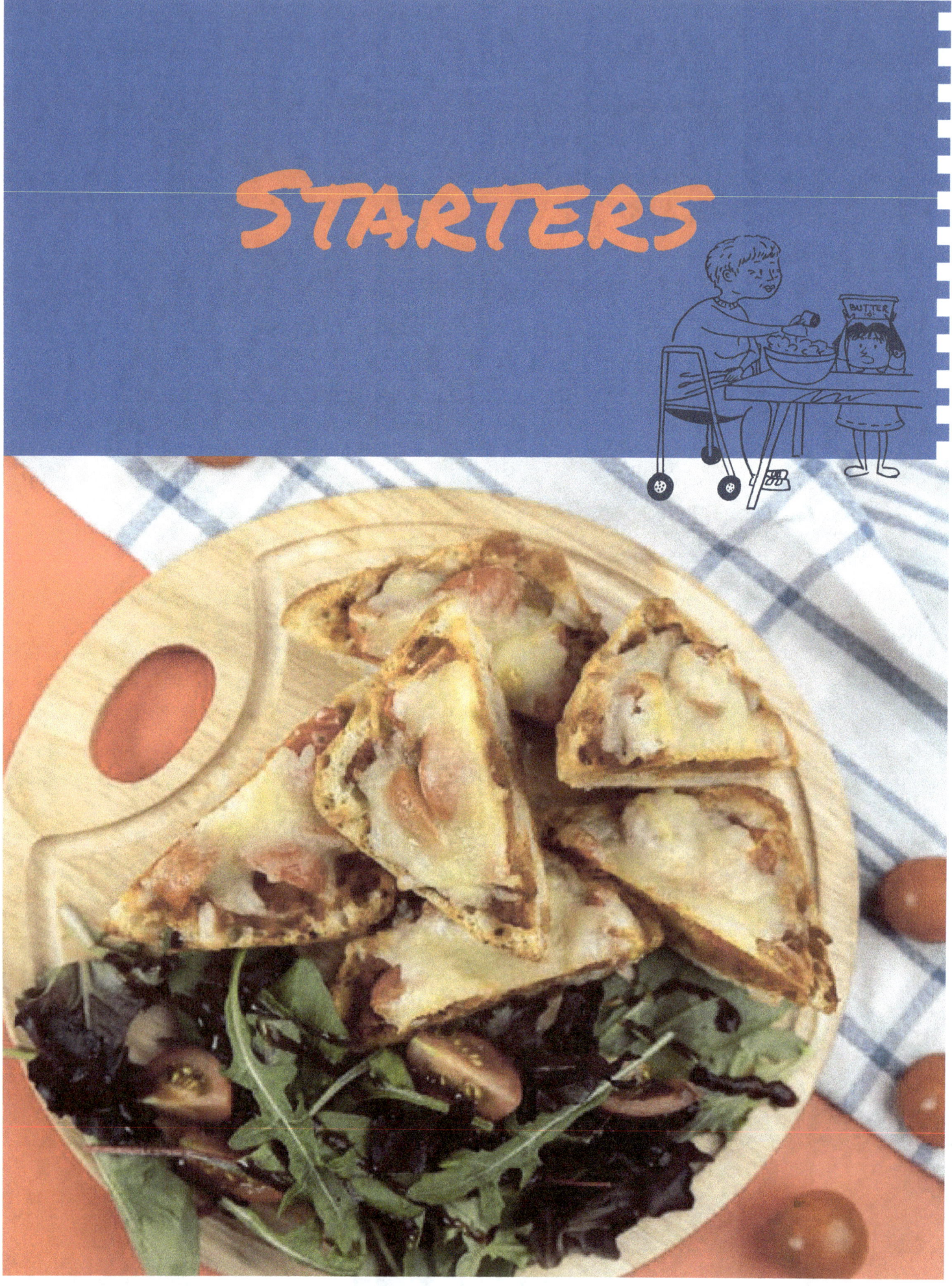

Cheesy Garlic Bread

Ingredients:

Par bake/bake at home bread • 1
Butter (softened) • 50g (2 tablespoons)
Easy garlic/garlic puree • 5mls (1 teaspoon)
Mozzarella or Mozzarella/Cheddar cheese (grated) • 50g

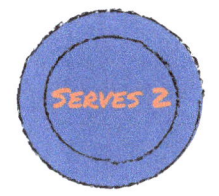

Serves 2

Method:

1. Set oven to Gas Mark 7, 220°C.
2. Make slits along the baguette (don't cut all the way through).
3. Make the garlic butter by mixing the softened butter with the garlic.
4. Mix the grated cheese and garlic butter together and divide evenly between the slits in the bread.
5. Place bread in a piece of tin foil – wrap up but leave top open to allow it to go golden brown.
6. Place in the hot oven for 10 minutes or until golden brown and butter has melted.

Cook's Tip: Buy ready-made garlic butter instead of making your own.

Why not try: Substitute the garlic butter and cheese mix for 'Boursin' garlic and herb cheese or try Dairylea cheese mixed with either some garlic powder or mixed herbs.

Sun-dried Tomato Rolls

Ingredients:

Bread Mix · 250g (½ a bag)
Sun-dried Tomatoes · 2
Warm water · 125mls (approx) to mix
Milk · for glazing

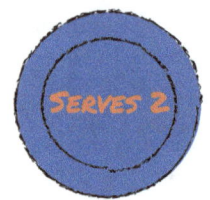

Serves 2

Method:

1. Set oven to Gas Mark 7, 220°C.
2. Place bread mix into a large bowl.
3. Cut up sun-dried tomatoes into small pieces with scissors and place into bowl with the bread mix.
4. Measure the warm water into a measuring jug.
5. Mix warm water into bread mix (a little at a time) to make a soft but not sticky dough.
6. Turn dough onto a lightly floured table top and knead until smooth.
7. Divide mixture into 4 equal pieces.
8. Knead each piece and form into a ball.
9. Place smooth side up on baking tray.
10. Cover with clingfilm and place in a warm place to rise for 10 minutes.
11. Remove clingfilm and brush lightly with milk.
12. Bake in a hot oven for 7-10 minutes until golden brown and sounds hollow when tapped.
13. Remove from oven and transfer to a cooling tray.

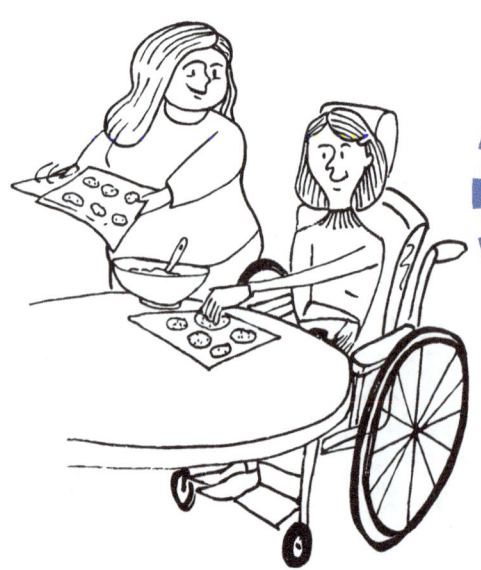

Cook's Tip:
The water needs to be lukewarm (you can touch it) to activate the yeast. It must NOT be boiling or cold.

Why Not Try:
Use olives instead of the sun-dried tomatoes

Add a chopped up Jalepeno Pepper to the mix with the sun-dried tomatoes to add a bit of spice.

Savoury Toasts

Ingredients:

Bloomer loaf • 4 slices
Onion • ¼ fresh medium OR 1 dessertsspoon frozen / fresh ready prepared chopped onion
Red Chilli • 2.5mls fresh finely chopped OR 2.5mls (1/2 teaspoon) frozen pre-chopped chilli
Garlic • 1 small clove (crushed) OR 2.5mls (½ teaspoons) frozen pre-chopped garlic or lazy/garlic puree
Cherry Tomatoes • 4
Pesto (red) • 30mls (2 tablespoons)
Parmesan cheese (grated) • 15mls
Oil • 5ml (1 teaspoon)

Serves 2

Method:

1. Set oven to Gas Mark 6, 200°C.
2. Peel and chop the onion and garlic if using fresh.
3. Roughly chop the tomatoes.
4. Heat oil in pan and sauté (gently fry) onion, garlic and chilli.
5. Add the chopped tomatoes and pesto.
6. Divide the mixture equally on to the top of the 4 slices of bread.
7. Sprinkle with the parmesan cheese and bake in the oven for 2-3 minutes until hot.

Why not try:

You can use grated Mozzarella or Mozzarella/Cheddar cheese instead of the Parmesan or you could combine the three types of cheese.

Chicken Filo Parcels

Ingredients:

Spring Onion • 1
Cooked Chicken • 2 slices
Tomato Puree • 5mls
Black Pepper to season
Butter • 50g (2 tablespoons)
Filo Pastry • 2 sheets

Method:

1. Set oven to Gas Mark 5, 190°C.
2. Wash, dry and finely chop spring onion to give a 15ml spoon.
3. Cut the chicken into small bits and mix with the spring onion and tomato puree.
4. Melt the butter and add a sprinkling of black pepper.
5. Divide the chicken mixture into 8 equal portions.
6. Cut the filo pastry into 8 rectangles, 6cm by 18cm and stack one on top of the other.

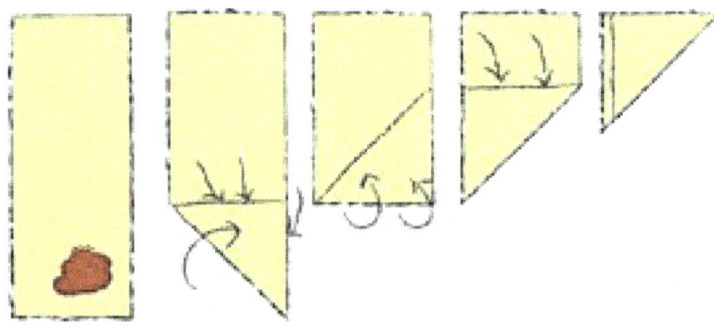

7. Lightly butter the edges of the top triangle. Place one of the chicken portions on the right hand side of the rectangle, closest to you (figure 1).
8. Fold the bottom left hand corner over the filling to make a triangle shape and seal the edges (figure 2).
9. Fold the right hand point up keeping the triangle shape and press in the edges to seal again.
10. Continue folding left then right sealing as you go until the end of the rectangle of pastry.
11. Place on a baking tray then repeat with the rest of the pastry.
12. Brush lightly with a little of the melted butter. Bake for 8 – 10 minutes until golden brown and serve with a sauce of your choice.

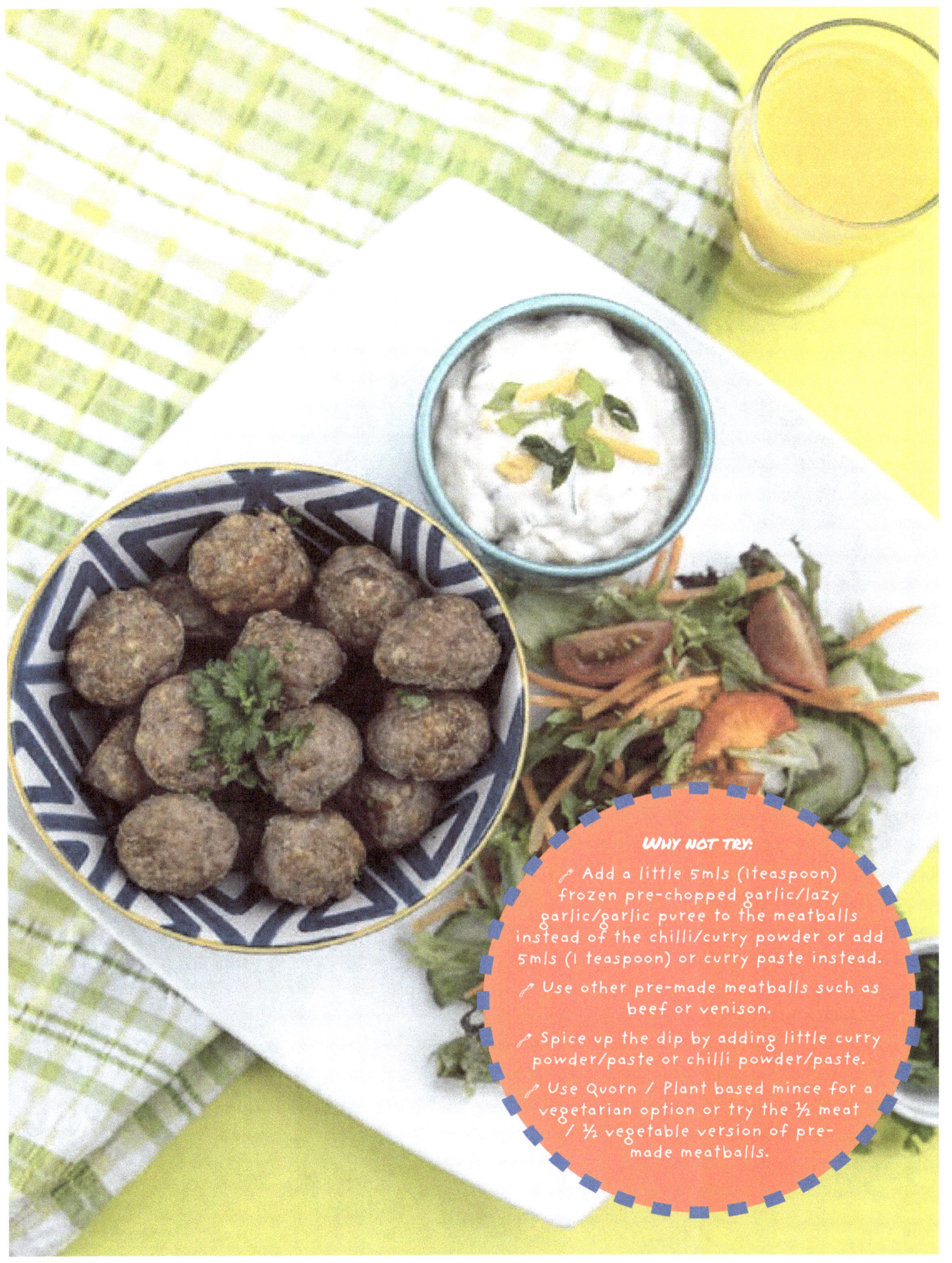

WHY NOT TRY:

- Add a little 5mls (1teaspoon) frozen pre-chopped garlic/lazy garlic/garlic puree to the meatballs instead of the chilli/curry powder or add 5mls (1 teaspoon) or curry paste instead.
- Use other pre-made meatballs such as beef or venison.
- Spice up the dip by adding little curry powder/paste or chilli powder/paste.
- Use Quorn / Plant based mince for a vegetarian option or try the ½ meat / ½ vegetable version of pre-made meatballs.

Turkey Meatballs with Cheese and Chive Dip

Ingredients:

Turkey Meatballs:
- **Turkey Mince** • 250g
- **Breadcrumbs** • 2 tablespoons
- **Beaten Egg** • 15mls (1 tablespoon)
- **Chilli or Curry powder** • Large pinch
- **Salt and pepper**

OR pre-prepared turkey meatballs

Dip:
- **Cream Cheese** • 15mls (1 tablespoon)
- **Natural Yoghurt** • 15mls (1 tablespoon)
- **Mayonnaise** • 15mls (1 tablespoon)
- **Chopped Chives** • 5mls (1 teaspoon)
- **Cheese (grated)** • 15mls (1 tablespoon)

Method:

1. To make the dip, start by placing all ingredients for dip in a clean bowl and blend using a wooden spoon or fork.
2. Place into serving dish.
3. If making your own meatballs, place all ingredients for meatballs into a bowl and mix with a fork.
4. Turn mixture out on to a clean board and divide into 12 equal portions.
5. Roll each piece into a ball using a little flour to prevent mixture sticking to hands.
6. Place on to a baking tray and bake in oven for 10 minutes until cooked all the way through.
7. Remove from baking tray and drain on kitchen paper.
8. Serve either hot or cold along with dip.

Tuna or Hot Smoked Salmon Pate with Toastie Soldiers

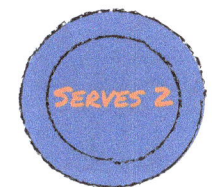
Serves 2

Ingredients:

Pate
- **Tuna** • 1 tin (drained) **OR** 2 fillets hot smoked salmon (skin removed)
- **Butter (softened)** • 50g (2 tablespoons)
- **Low fat Cream Cheese** • 50g
- **Lemon Juice** • 15mls (1 tablespoon)
- **Black Pepper**

Toastie Soldiers
- **Wholemeal or White Bread** • 4 slices

Garnish
- **Lemon twists & sprigs of parsley**

Serving Suggestions:

Serve with a little green salad and a drizzle of Balsamic Dressing.
Serve a basket of additional toastie soldiers with the pate.

Method:

1. **Pate:**
   Open the tin of tuna and drain thoroughly (see tip below) or using a fork flake the hot smoked salmon.

2. Place drained tuna or flaked salmon, butter, cream cheese, and lemon juice into a processor and blend until smooth (see tip below).

3. Add pepper and more lemon juice if required to taste.

4. Divide the mixture between 4 small individual ramekin dishes and level the surface.

5. Cover and chill for 30 minutes.

6. Serve with lemon twists and parsley.

   Toastie Soldiers:

7. Toast the bread in a toaster or under the grill.

8. Remove the crusts from the bread if you can.

9. Cut each slice of toast into 3 fingers.

10. Serve on a clean plate beside the ramekin of pate.

Cook's Tip:
- Drain the tuna using a sieve.
- If you don't have a food processor then place the mixture into a jug and blend with a hand blender or a fork.

Fish Goujons with Tomato Salsa

Serves 2

Ingredients:

Fish (eg. haddock / smoked haddock / salmon / trout) – 2 fillets
Breadcrumbs • 4 tablespoons
Cajun seasoning • 2.5mls (½ teaspoon)
Beaten Egg • 1 egg
Plain Flour • 25g (1 tablespoon)
Oil for greasing tray

Method:

1. Put oven on to Gas Mark 6, 200°C.
2. Mix the breadcrumbs (see tip below) with the Cajun seasoning in a bowl.
3. Beat the egg in a small bowl and season with a little salt and pepper.
4. Place the flour on to a plate.
5. Cut the fish into even sized strips removing any bones.
6. Coat each piece of fish in the flour then dip in the egg and then the breadcrumbs.
7. Place on to a greased baking tray and bake in the oven for 10-15 minutes.
8. Remove from oven and serve with tomato salsa.

Why not try:

- Use thin strips of chicken instead of fish.
- Use Quorn / Plant based pieces for a vegetarian option.
- Use spray oil to grease the tray.
- Use Natural (Panco) breadcrumbs instead of making your own.

Bruschetta

Ingredients:

Par bake/bake at home bread · 2 small or 4 slices of garlic bread/ Ciabattas slices
Pesto (red) · 30mls (2 tablespoons)
Cheddar or Mozzarella cheese (grated) · 75g (3 tablespoons)
Cherry tomatoes · 4

Serves 2

Serving Suggestions:

Use chopped peppers and/or salami/ham/chorizo/plant based alternative etc, to improve the nutritional value, colour, flavour and texture.

Drizzle a little Balsamic glaze over the salad leaves.

Method:

1. Set oven to Gas Mark 6, 200°C.
2. Place the garlic bread slices / ciabattas or baked baguettes (cut in half lengthwise if using).
3. Spread the pesto thinly over each slice of the bread.
4. Slice the tomatoes in quarters.
5. Place the tomatoes over the pesto.
6. Sprinkle the cheese on the top of each bruschetta being careful not to drop the cheese onto the tray as this will burn in the oven.
7. Place the tray in the oven and bake for 5 minutes or until the cheese has melted.
8. Take out and place on a clean plate and garnish with a few salad leaves and wedges of tomato.

Tomato Salsa

Ingredients:

Tomatoes (firm) - 2 large
Red Onion - ¼ (diced) **OR** 1 dessertspoon frozen/fresh pre-diced red onion
Lime - ½
Coriander - 2.5mls (1/2 teaspoon) of fresh / frozen chopped **OR** 1.2mls dried coriander
Olive Oil - 5mls

Serves 2

Serving Suggestions:

Serve with the cheese and chive dip from the Turkey Meatballs recipe.

Method:

1. Wash tomatoes then chop and place in a bowl.
2. Wash, peel and finely chop or grate the red onion and add to the tomatoes.
3. Grate the zest of the lime and add to the tomatoes along with 5mls of the juice to the bowl with the onions and tomato.
4. Add the olive oil.
5. Roughly chop the coriander if using fresh.
6. Add coriander to the bowl. Stir mixture through and serve with the fish goujons.

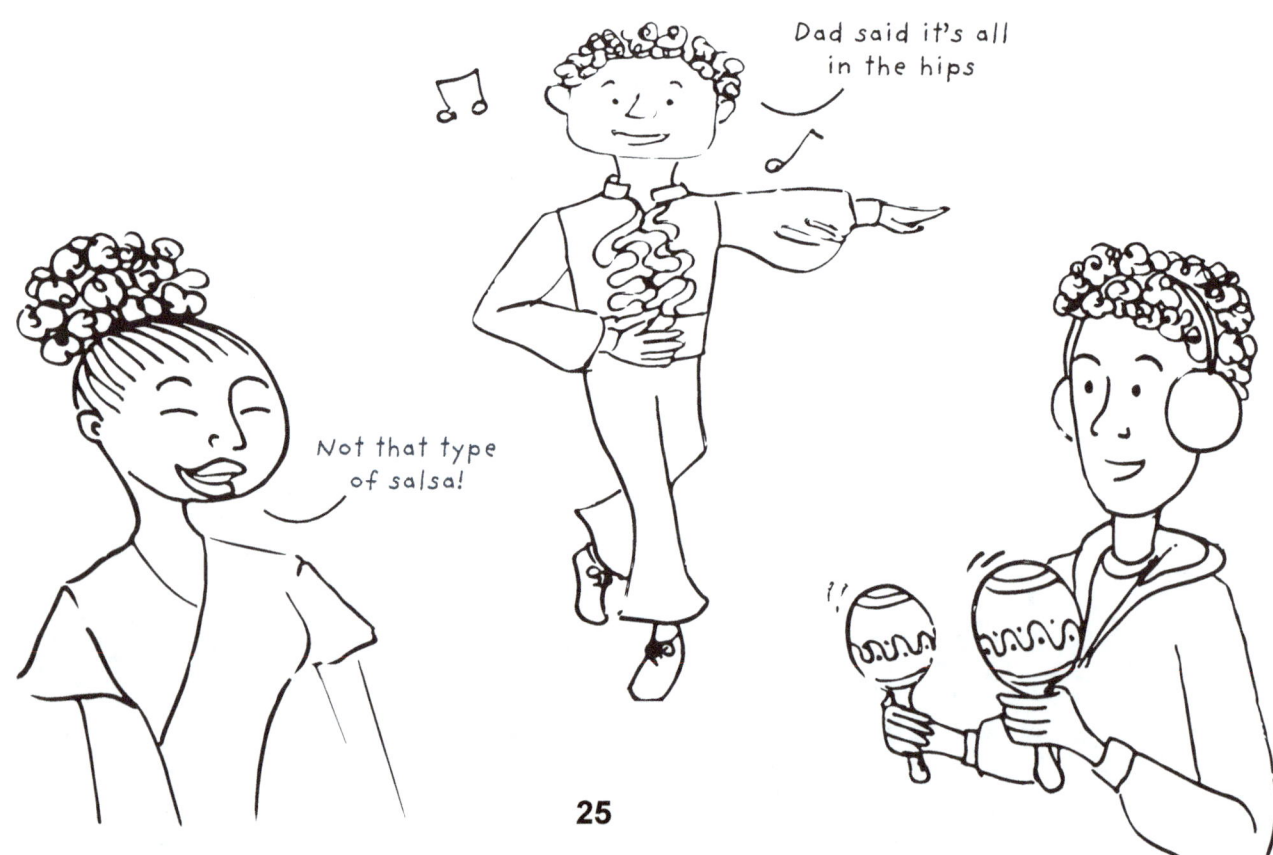

SOUPS

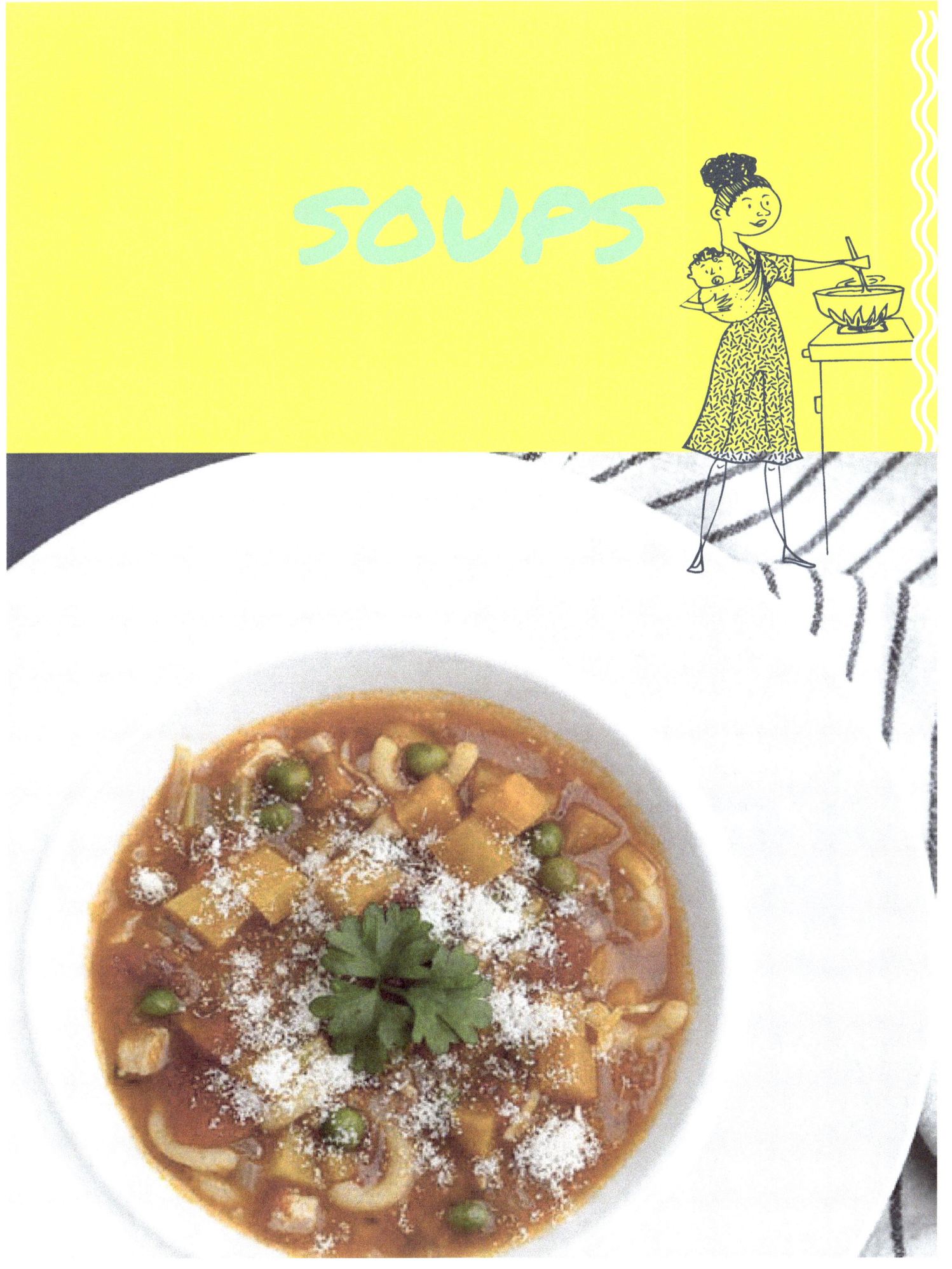

Tomato, Lentil, & Red Pepper Soup

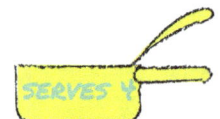
Serves 4

Ingredients:

Oil · 5ml (1 teaspoon)
Onion · 1 medium fresh **OR** 100g (3 tablespoons) frozen / fresh ready prepared chopped onion
Garlic · 1 clove (crushed) **OR** 5mls (1 teaspoons) frozen pre-chopped garlic **OR** lazy/garlic puree
Red peppers · 2 fresh **OR** 150g ready prepared or frozen mixed peppers
Chopped tomatoes · 1 large tin (450ml)
Lentils · 150g (1 mug)
Vegetable stock cubes or stock pots · 2
Water · 500mls (1 pint)
Parsley · small fresh bunch (chopped) **OR** 10mls (2 teaspoons) frozen pre-chopped parsley

Method:

1. Prepare the vegetables as follows if using fresh:
   - Peel and roughly chop the onion
   - Wash, remover seeds and roughly chop the red pepper
   - Peel and crush the garlic
2. Heat the oil in a pan, add the onion, garlic and red pepper. Cook gently for 5 minutes stirring with a wooden spoon.
3. Add the tomatoes, lentils, stock cubes/pots and water.
4. Bring to the boil and simmer for 10 minutes with the lid on.
5. Blend the soup using an electric hand blender or liquidiser.
6. Taste for seasoning
7. Reheat soup and serve.

Cream of Lentil Soup with Croutons

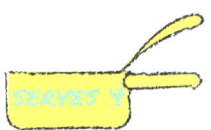
Serves 4

Ingredients:

Onion · 1 medium fresh **OR** 100g (3 tablespoons) frozen / fresh ready prepared chopped onion
Carrot · 2 large fresh **OR** 400g (4 mugs) ready prepared fresh carrot batons / 1/3 bag of frozen sliced carrots
Turnip · ¼ fresh **OR** 100g (1 mug) ready prepared turnip peeled and diced
Vegetable stock cubes or stock pots · 2
Water · 1 litre (2 pints)
Lentils · 150g (1 mug)
Single Cream · 100mls (1/3 of a mug)
Salt and Pepper
Parsley · small fresh bunch (chopped) **OR** 10mls (2 teaspoons) frozen pre-chopped parsley

COOK'S TIP: Use the crustless bread for making the croutons or buy ready-made croutons.

Method:

1. Prepare the vegetables as follows if using fresh:
   - Onion – peel and roughly chop
   - Carrot – peel and roughly chop
   - Turnip – peel and roughly chop
2. Place stock, lentils, and vegetables in large pan and bring to the boil.
3. Simmer for 30 minutes until vegetables are soft.
4. Remove from heat and puree using a hand blender/liquidiser or use a potato masher for a chunkier soup.
5. Stir in cream and check seasoning.
6. Sprinkle chopped parsley over top to serve.

Croutons

Ingredients:

Bread · 2 – 3 slices
Spray oil

Method:

1. Remove crusts from bread and cut into small cubes (1cm cube)
2. Spray or brush a baking tray with oil.
3. Spread cubes of bread over tray then spray bread with oil.
4. Bake in a hot oven (Gas Mark 7, 210'C) for 5 minutes until golden brown and crisp.

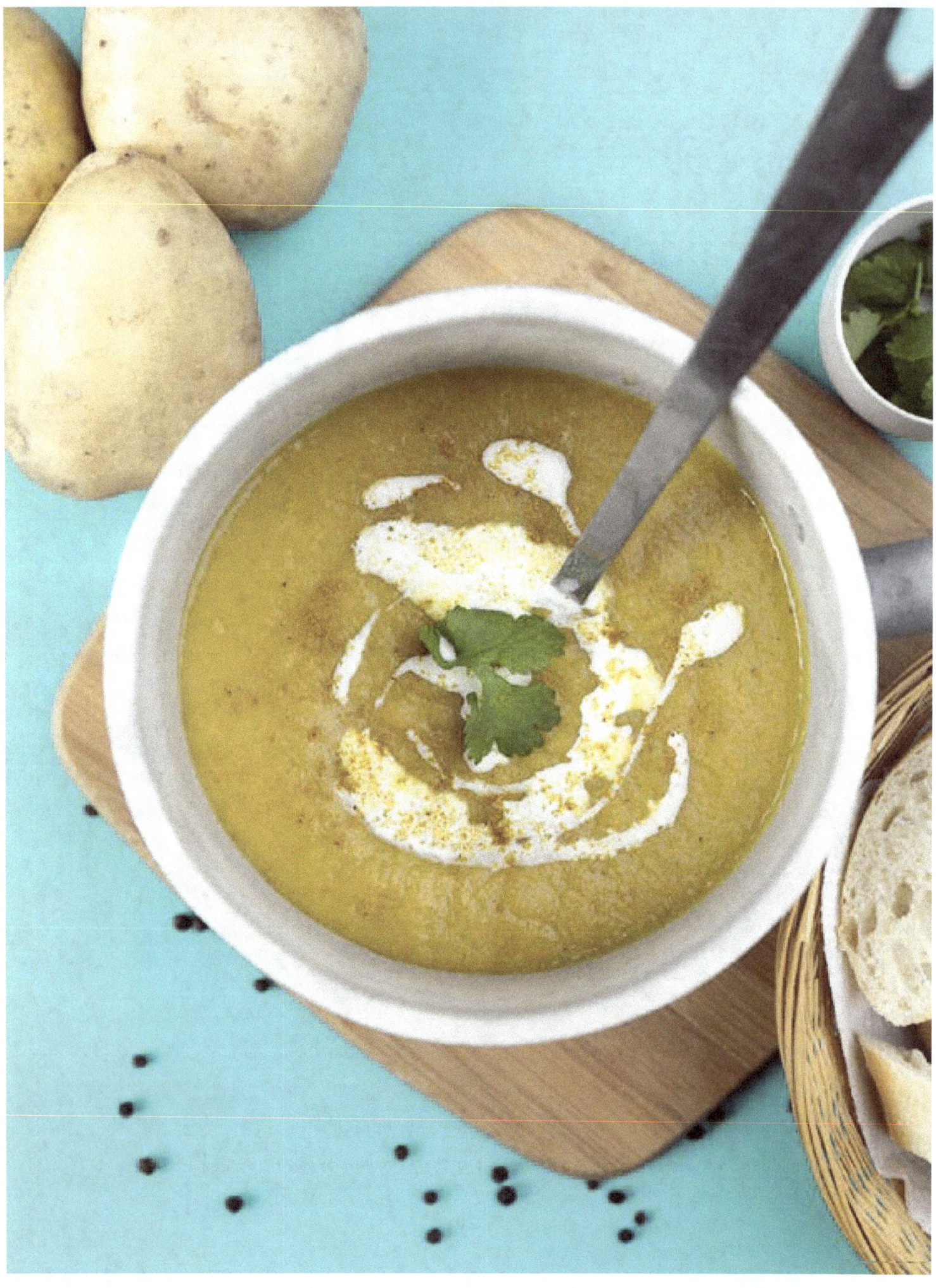

Spicy Leek and Potato Soup

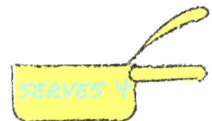

Ingredients:

Leek · 1 large **OR** 300g frozen pre-sliced leek
Onion · 1 medium fresh **OR** 100g (3 tablespoons) frozen / fresh ready prepared chopped onion
Potatoes · 4 medium sized fresh (approx. 250g)
Oil · 15ml (1 tablespoon)
Curry paste · 5 to 10mls (1 to 2 teaspoons)
Vegetable stock cubes or stock pots · 2
Single Cream · 100mls (1/3 of a mug)
Salt and pepper
Parsley · small fresh bunch (chopped) **OR** 10mls (2 teaspoons) frozen pre-chopped parsley

Method:

1. Measure / prepare the following ingredients if using fresh:
   - Leek – wash and roughly slice
   - Onion – peel and roughly chop
   - Potatoes – peel and roughly chop
   - Stock – dissolve stock cubes/pots in 500mls boiling water

2. Heat oil in large pan and sauté vegetables with the oil and curry paste for 2-3 minutes.

3. Add the stock cubes/stock pots and water and bring to the boil.

4. Simmer for 25-20 minutes until vegetables are tender.

5. Remove from heat and puree using a hand blender/liquidiser or use a potato masher for a chunkier soup.

6. Stir in cream and check seasoning.

7. Sprinkle chopped parsley over top to serve.

Butternut Squash & Sweet Potato Soup

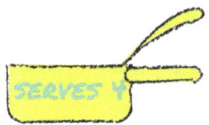
SERVES 4

Ingredients:

Oil · 10ml (1 dessertspoon)
Garlic · 1 clove (crushed) OR 5mls (1 teaspoons) frozen pre-chopped garlic OR lazy/garlic puree
Onion · 1 medium fresh OR 100g (3 tablespoons) frozen / fresh ready prepared chopped onion
Carrot · 1 small fresh OR 100g (1 mug) ready prepared diced carrot / ¼ bag frozen sliced carrots
Lentils · 75g (½ mug)
Water · 1 litre (2 pints)
Sweet Potato · 300g fresh OR frozen/ready prepared sweet potato
Butternut Squash · 1 small fresh OR 500g frozen/ready prepared sweet potato
Vegetable stock cubes or stock pots · 2 cubes
Curry or Chilli powder · 5ml (1 teaspoon) if you wish to make it spicy (optional)
Crème Fraiche or Cream · 30 ml (optional)
Salt and pepper
Parsley · small fresh bunch (chopped) or 10mls (2 teaspoons) frozen pre-chopped parsley

Method:

1. Prepare the vegetables as follows if using fresh:
   - Peel the carrot, sweet potato, and butternut squash then roughly chop.
   - Peel and dice the onion.
   - Peel and crush the garlic.

2. On a medium heat add oil to the pan and gently fry the onion and garlic together with the lid on for about 2 minutes until the onion softens (do not brown).

3. Add the carrot, sweet potato, butternut squash, lentils (and spices if using) and cook gently for about 5 minutes — stirring all the time.

4. Add the stock cubes/stock pots and water. Bring to the boil then reduce the heat and simmer for 15-20 minutes with the lid on, or until all vegetables are tender.

5. Either:
   - leave the soup as it is.
   - blend the soup with a hand blender.
6. - mash with a potato masher.

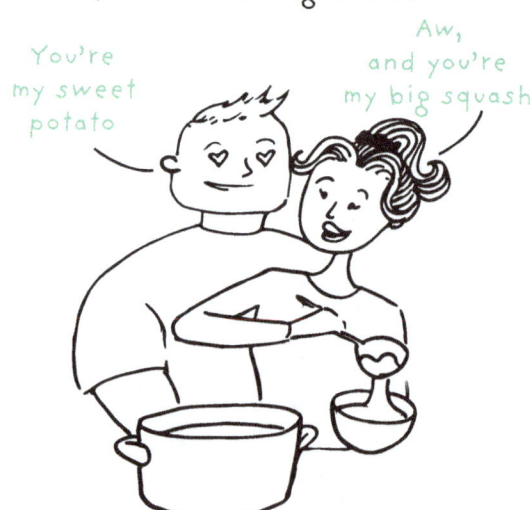

Carrot & Sweet Potato Soup

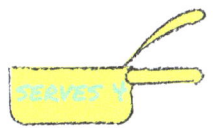

Ingredients:

Onion · 1 medium fresh **OR** 100g (3 tablespoons) frozen / fresh ready prepared chopped onion
Carrot · 2 large fresh **OR** 400g (4 mugs) ready prepared fresh carrot batons / 1/3 bag of frozen sliced carrots
Sweet potato · 300g fresh (approx. 2 large) **OR** frozen/ready prepared sweet potato
Vegetable stock cubes or stock pots · 2
Water · 1 litre (2 pints)
Coriander (ground) · 5ml (1 teaspoon)
Oil · 5ml (1 teaspoon)
Crème Fraiche or Cream · 30 ml (optional)
Salt and pepper
Parsley · small fresh bunch (chopped) **OR** 10mls (2 teaspoons) frozen pre-chopped parsley

Method:

1. Prepare the vegetables as follows if using fresh:
   - Wash, peel and roughly chop the carrots.
   - Wash, peel and roughly chop the sweet potato
   - Peel and roughly chop the onion.

2. Heat the oil in a pan, add the onion, carrot and sweet potato and cook gently for 5 minutes, stirring all the time.

3. Add the water, stock cubes/pots, dried coriander and bring to the boil.

4. Simmer with a lid on for 20 minutes or until the vegetables are soft.

5. Leave to cool slightly then blend with a hand blender / liquidiser.

6. Add the crème fraiche, taste and season with salt and pepper.

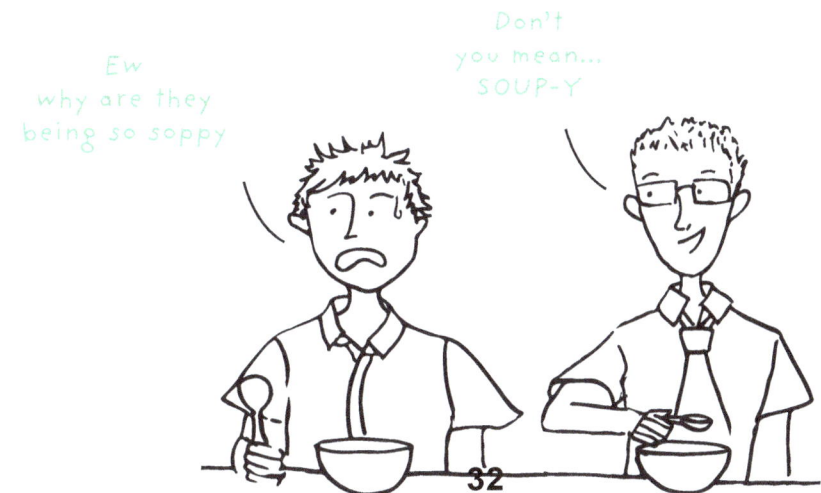

Tomato & Bean Soup

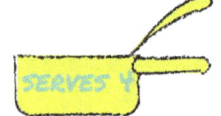

Ingredients:

Margarine · 12.5g (2 teaspoons)
Onion · ½ medium fresh **OR** 50g (2 tablespoons) frozen / fresh ready prepared chopped onion
Carrot · 1 small fresh **OR** 100g (1 mug) ready prepared fresh carrot batons / ¼ bag of frozen sliced carrots
Butter Beans (drained) · 1 small tin (200mls)
Chopped tomatoes · 1 small tin (200ml)
Vegetable stock cubes or stock pots · 1
Dried Thyme · 1.25mls (¼ teaspoon)
Sugar · Pinch

Method:

1. Prepare vegetables as follows if using fresh:
   - Onion – peel and finely chop
   - Carrot – peel and grate

2. Measure water into a jug and add stock cube/stock pot.

3. Place tinned tomatoes into jug with stock.

4. Add thyme and sugar to jug with stock and tomatoes.

5. Drain beans.

6. Place carrot, onion and margarine into a pan and sauté (lightly fry) until they have started to soften, do not brown.

7. Remove from heat and add the contents from the jug and the butter beans.

8. Simmer for 20 minutes.

9. Remove from heat and season to taste. Serve.

Carrot & Courgette Soup

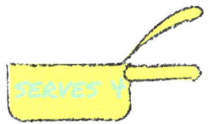

Ingredients:

Onion · 1 medium fresh **OR** 100g (3 tablespoons) frozen / fresh ready prepared chopped onion
Courgettes · 2 medium fresh
Carrot · 3 small fresh **OR** 300g (3 mugs) ready prepared fresh carrot batons ½ bag of frozen sliced carrots
Boiling Water · 1 litre (2 pints)
Vegetable stock cubes or stock pots · 2
Margarine · 25g (1 tablespoon)
Parsley · small fresh bunch (chopped) **OR** 10mls (2 teaspoons) frozen pre-chopped parsley

Method:

1. Prepare vegetables as follows if using fresh:
   - Onion – Peel and chop.
   - Courgette – wash and roughly slice.
   - Carrot – Peel and roughly slice.

2. Melt margarine in pan and add vegetables.

3. Sauté (gently fry) for 2 minutes.

4. Add water and stock cubes/pots.

5. Bring to the boil, cover with a lid and simmer until vegetables are soft.

6. Remove from heat and blend or use a potato masher for a chunkier soup.

7. Check for seasoning then serve with finely chopped parsley.

Tomato & Basil Soup

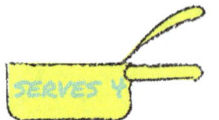

Ingredients:

Onion · 1 medium fresh or 100g (3 tablespoons) frozen / fresh ready prepared chopped onion
Carrot · 1 small fresh or 100g (1 mug) ready prepared diced carrot / ¼ bag frozen sliced carrots
Garlic · 1 clove (crushed) or 5mls (1 teaspoons) frozen pre-chopped garlic or lazy/garlic puree
Oil · 15ml (1 tablespoon)
Chopped tomatoes · 1 large tin (450ml)
Vegetable stock cubes or stock pots · 2
Celery · ½ stalk washed and sliced (optional)
Fresh Tomatoes · 2 washed and roughly chopped
Basil · 2.5mls (1/2 teaspoon) either fresh or pre-frozen
Sugar · 2.5mls (1/2 teaspoon)
Black pepper to season
Basil · small fresh bunch (chopped) or 10mls (2 teaspoons) frozen pre-chopped basil

Method:

1. Prepare vegetables as follows if using fresh:
   - Onion – Peel and chop
   - Carrot – Peel and roughly slice
   - Garlic – Peel and roughly chop or crush
   - Celery – washed and sliced

2. Wash and roughly chop the fresh tomatoes.

3. Heat oil in pan, add onion, garlic, carrot and celery and sweat (cook very gently on a low heat) with lid on for 3-4 minutes to soften.

4. Add stock cubes/pots, 300mls water, tinned tomatoes, basil, sugar and black pepper to the pan.

5. Bring to the boil.

6. Add the fresh tomatoes to the pan and simmer with the lid on for 15 minutes.

7. Remove from heat, blend and season to taste.

Cook's Tip: Add a handful of roughly chopped basil leaves and 15mls cream prior to blending.

Mushroom, Sweet Potato, & Carrot Soup

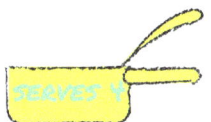

Ingredients:

Oil · 5ml (1 teaspoon)
Onion · 1 medium fresh **OR** 100g (3 tablespoons) frozen / fresh ready prepared chopped onion
Sweet potato · 300g fresh (approx. 2 large) **OR** frozen/ready prepared sweet potato
Mushrooms · 250g fresh **OR** frozen/ready prepared **OR** 2 cans of tinned mushrooms
Carrot · 1 small fresh **OR** 100g (1 mug) ready prepared diced carrot / ¼ bag frozen sliced carrots
Lentils · 75g (½ mug)
Cumin (ground) · 2.5 to 5 ml (1/2 – 1 teaspoon)
Coriander (ground) · 2.5ml (1/2 teaspoon)
Cornflour · 15ml (1 level tablespoon)
Vegetable stock cubes OR stock pots · 2
Water · 1 litre (2 pints)
Crème Fraiche OR Cream · 30 ml (optional)
Salt and pepper

Garnish
Parsley · small fresh bunch (chopped) **OR** 10mls (2 teaspoons) frozen pre-chopped parsley

Serving Suggestions:

Garnish with chopped parsley. Serve with hot garlic or crusty bread.

Method:

1. Prepare the vegetables as follows if using fresh:
   - Peel and roughly chop the onion
   - Wash, peel and roughly chop the sweet potato and carrot
   - Wash and slice or chop the mushrooms

2. Heat the oil, add the onion, cumin, coriander and cornflour, and gently fry for 2 minutes.

3. Add the rest of the vegetables, lentils and stock cube/stock pot and the water.

4. Bring to the boil and simmer for 20-30 minutes until the vegetables are soft.

5. Blend or mash with a potato masher.

6. Taste for seasoning.

7. Stir in the crème fraiche or cream if using and serve.

Minestrone Soup

Ingredients:

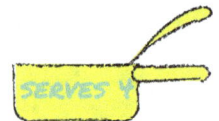

Onion · 1 medium fresh **OR** 100g (3 tablespoons) frozen / fresh ready prepared chopped onion
Carrot · 1 large fresh **OR** 200g (2 mugs) ready prepared fresh carrot batons / ½ bag of frozen sliced carrots
Turnip · ¼ fresh **OR** 100g (1 mug) ready prepared turnip peeled and diced
Celery · 1 stalk (sliced)
Cabbage · 50g sliced or ½ a mug of frozen pre-shredded savoy cabbage
Frozen Peas · 50g (3 tablesoons)
Garlic · 2 cloves (crushed) or 10mls (2 teaspoons) frozen pre-chopped garlic **OR** lazy/ garlic puree
Lardons · 1 small pack (unsmoked)
Chopped tomatoes · 1 large tin (450ml)
Vegetable stock cubes or stock pots · 2
Sugar · 2.5mls (1 level teaspoon)
Spaghetti · 30g **OR** small pasta for soup eg. Macaroni, Shells, Orzo,
Oil · 15ml (1 tablespoon)

Garnish
Parsley · small fresh bunch (chopped) **OR** 10mls (2 teaspoons) frozen pre-chopped parsley
Parmesan (grated) · 20mls (4 teaspoons)

Serving suggestions:

Sprinkle a little grated parmesan over the top and garnish with parsley.
Serve with hot garlic or crusty bread.

Method:

1. Measure / prepare the following ingredients if using fresh:
   - Onion – peel and dice
   - Garlic – peel and crush
   - Carrot – peel and dice
   - Turnip – peel and dice
   - Celery – wash and slice
   - Cabbage – wash and shred
   - Parsley – wash and chop
   - Spaghetti – break into 2cm pieces (see tip below)
   - Stock – dissolve stock cubes/pots in 500mls boiling water

2. Heat the oil in a large deep pan and gently sauté (lightly fry with the lid on) the onion, lardons and garlic until soft – do not allow to go brown.

3. Add the carrot, turnip and celery to the pot and sauté for a further minute, again without colouring

4. Add the tinned tomatoes, stock and sugar to the pot and bring to the boil

5. Add a little salt and pepper then place lid on pot and simmer for 10 minutes.

6. Add spaghetti and cook for a further 10 minutes.

7. Add cabbage and peas and cook for a further 5 minutes

8. Taste soup and adjust seasoning if required.

9. Transfer to a serving dish and sprinkle with parsley.

COOK'S TIP:
To prepare the spaghetti – roll up long ways in a tea towel. Hold each end of the tea towel and pull down the edge of the work surface a couple of times to break the spaghetti.

Lentil, Carrot, & Apple Soup

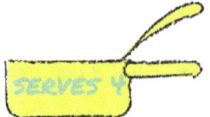

Ingredients:

Onion · 1 medium fresh **OR** 100g (3 tablespoons) frozen / fresh ready prepared chopped onion
Carrot · 2 large fresh **OR** 400g (4 mugs) ready prepared fresh carrot batons / 1/3 bag of frozen sliced carrots
Cooking Apple · 1 medium (100g)
Lentils · 75g (½ mug)
Oil · 10ml (1 dessertspoon)
Curry Powder (medium) · 10ml (2 teaspoons)
Ham stock cubes or stock pots · 2
Water · 1 litre (2 pints)
Salt and pepper

Garnish
Parsley · small fresh bunch (chopped) **OR** 10mls (2 teaspoons) frozen pre-chopped parsley

Method:

1. Prepare ingredients as follows if using fresh:
   - Wash, peel, and roughly chop the carrot.
   - Peel and roughly chop the onion.
   - Peel and roughly chop the apple.
2. Heat the oil in a large pan.
3. Add the onion and gently cook for 2 minutes with lid on, do not brown.
4. Add the curry powder and stir to coat the onion, cook for 1 minute.
5. Add the lentils, carrot and apple to the pan.
6. Add the stock cubes/pots and the water.
7. Bring to the boil and simmer for 20 minutes or until the carrots are soft.
8. Cool the soup slightly and puree using a hand blender or liquidiser.
9. Taste the soup for seasoning, reheat and serve.

SPICY LENTIL SOUP

INGREDIENTS:

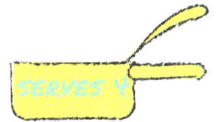

Lentils · 75g (½ mug)
Carrot · 1 large fresh **OR** 200g (2 mugs) ready prepared fresh carrot batons / ¼ bag of frozen sliced carrots
Onion · 1 medium fresh **OR** 100g (3 tablespoons) frozen / fresh ready prepared chopped onion
Turnip · ¼ fresh **OR** 100g (1 mug) ready prepared turnip peeled and diced
Vegetable or ham stock cubes OR stock pots · 1
Water · 1 litre (2 pints)
Potatoes · 4 medium sized fresh (approx. 250g)
Kidney Beans (tinned) · 50g (2 tablespoons)
Chilli Powder · 5ml (1 teaspoon)

Optional:
Cumin · pinch
Coriander · pinch   } These can be added for a slightly spicier soup
Garam Masala · pinch

Crème Fraiche or Cream · 30mls (2 tablespoons) – Optional
Garnish
Parsley · small fresh bunch (chopped) **OR** 10mls (2 teaspoons) frozen pre-chopped parsley

SERVING SUGGESTION:

If you want to make it creamy add the single cream or crème fraiche at step 6. Serve garnished with parsley if wished.

METHOD:

1. Add the lentils, stock cube and water into a pan and bring to the boil.
2. Prepare the vegetables as follows if using fresh:
   - Wash, peel the carrot. Grate using a food processor or grater.
   - Wash and peel the turnip. Grate using a food processor or grater.
   - Wash and dice the potato – no need to peel
3. Peel the onion and finely chop
4. Add the vegetables to the soup
5. Add the chilli powder.
6. Add the cumin, coriander and garam masala if using.
7. Bring to the boil and simmer for 10 minutes with the lid on.
8. Add the kidney beans and bring back to the boil.
9. Taste for seasoning.

Sweet Potato & Mixed Pepper Soup

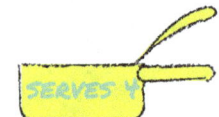

Ingredients:

Sweet potato · 250g (prepared weight) — fresh or frozen
Potato · 150g (prepared weight)
Mixed Peppers · 75g fresh or frozen
Onion · 1 medium fresh **OR** 100g (3 tablespoons) frozen / fresh ready prepared chopped onion
Garlic · 1 clove (crushed) **OR** 5mls (1 teaspoons) frozen pre-chopped garlic or lazy/garlic puree
Oil · 10ml (1 dessertspoon)
Vegetable stock cubes or stock pots · 2
Water · 1 litre (2 pints)

Garnish
Parsley · small fresh bunch (chopped) **OR** 10mls (2 teaspoons) frozen pre-chopped parsley

Method:

1. Wash, peel and roughly chop both potatoes if using fresh.
2. Roughly chop the pepper if using fresh.
3. Heat the oil in a large pan, add the onion and peppers and saute on a low heat with the lid on for approximately 5 minutes until soft but not brown.
4. Add the garlic and cook for a further minute.
5. Add the potatoes, vegetable stock cubes/pots and water.
6. Bring to the boil, cover and simmer for 20 minutes until the potatoes are tender.
7. Allow the soup to cool slightly before blending using a hand blender or liquidiser.
8. Reheat the soup adjust the consistency and seasoning if necessary.
9. Serve.

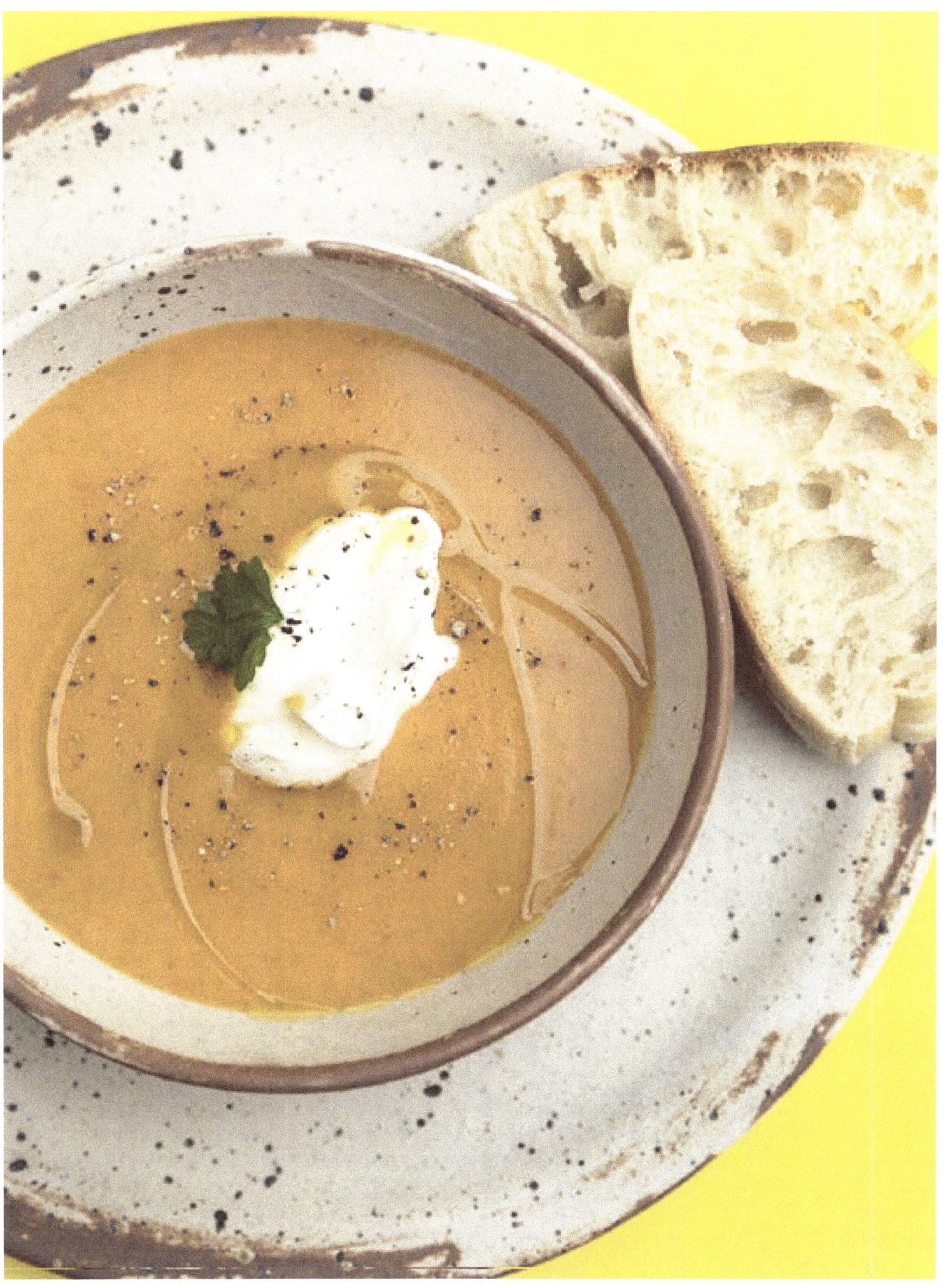

MAINS

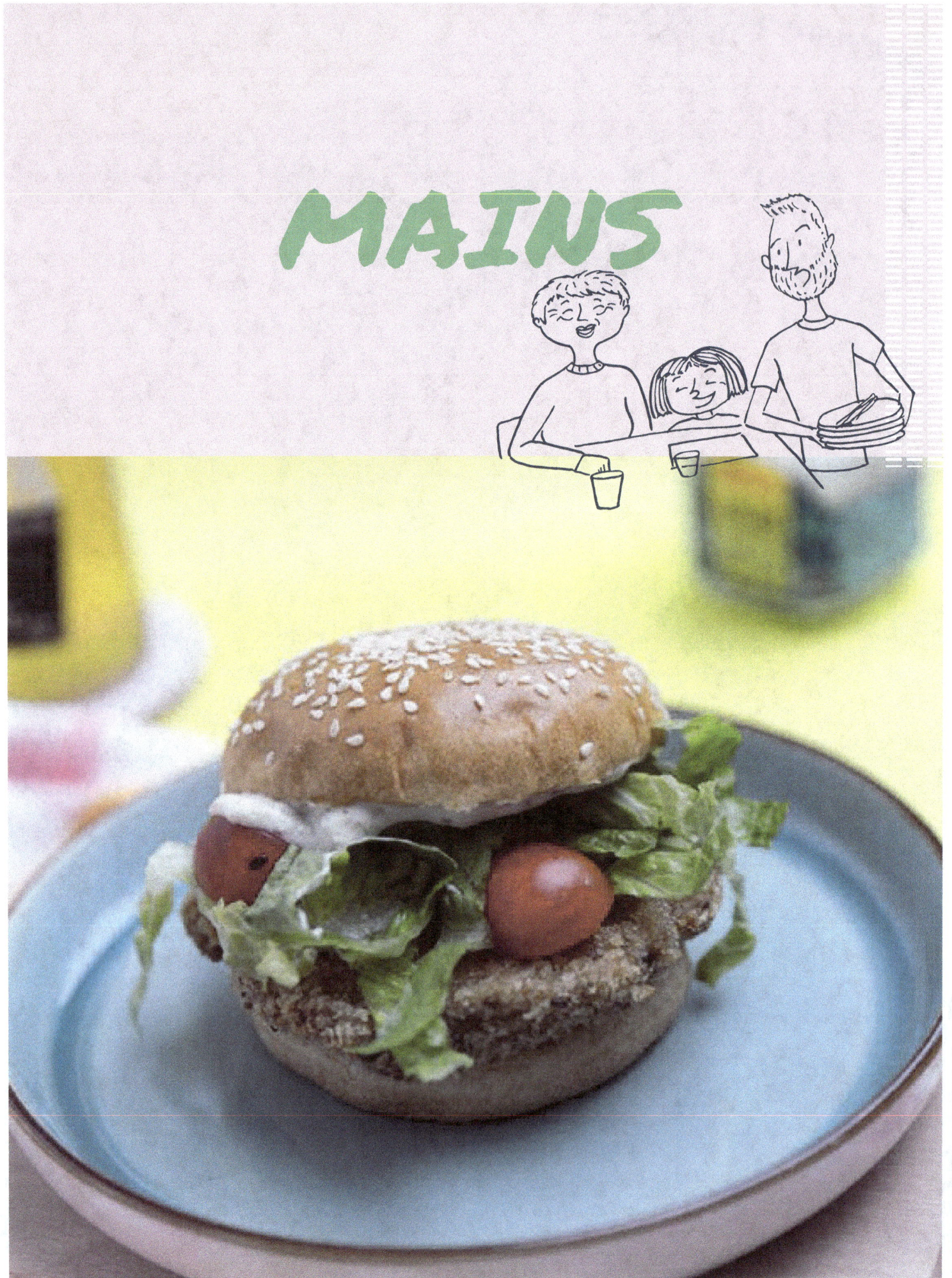

Chilli Con Carne

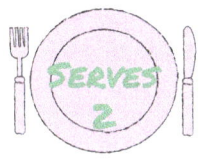

Ingredients:

Onion   1 small fresh or 50g (2 tablespoons) frozen/fresh ready prepared diced onion
Red/Green Pepper   ½ fresh or 50g (2 tablespoons) ready prepared or frozen mixed peppers
Minced Beef   250g fresh or frozen
Chilli Powder   2.5mls (½ teaspoon)
Beef stock cubes/stock pots/Oxo   1 dissolved in 150mls (½ a mug) boiling water
Chopped Tomatoes (tinned)   1 small tin (200ml) or ½ large tin
Tomato Puree   15mls (1 level tablespoon)
Kidney Beans in Chilli Sauce   1 small tin or ½ large tin
Tomato Ketchup   5mls (1 teaspoon)
Sugar   Pinch
Long Grain Rice   300g (2 mugs) or 2 packets microwave rice / 4 packs frozen microwaveable rice
Salt & Pepper

Method:

1. Prepare ingredients as follows if using fresh:
   - Peel and chop the onion
   - Wash, deseed, and chop the pepper

2. Make up the stock and add tinned tomatoes, tomato puree, tomato sauce, sugar, chilli and chilli beans to jug with stock.

3. Place mince into a pan and cook on a high heat, stirring all the time until the mince has broken up and turned brown.

4. Stir in the onion and peppers.

5. Add the rest of the ingredients from the jug and a little salt and pepper to the pan and bring to simmering point. Put lid on the pan and simmer gently for about 20 minutes until the mince is cooked.

6. Half fill another pan with water, add salt and bring to the boil.

7. When water is boiling add rice and simmer, stirring occasionally until cooked.

8. Drain the rice through a sieve, rinse with boiling water and place into a warm ovenproof dish. (Alternatively prepare the microwave rice according to the instructions on the packet.)

9. Remove the chilli from the heat and season to taste (add more chilli powder at this stage if you want it spicier)

10. Make a nest in the rice and spoon the chilli mixture carefully into the centre and serve.

Cheesy Tuna Fishcakes

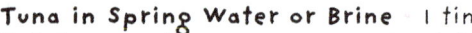

Ingredients:

Tuna in Spring Water or Brine 1 tin
Potatoes 2 large or 425g pack of fresh pre-mashed potatoes
Parsley 5mls (1 teaspoon) finely chopped frozen or fresh
Butter 5g (1 teaspoon)
Grated Cheese 25g (1 tablespoon)
Milk 10mls (1 dessertspoon) if using fresh potatoes and required
Salt and Pepper
Egg 1 beaten
Plain Flour 25g (1 tablespoon)
Natural/Panko Breadcrumbs 1 cup (½ mug) (see tip below) or Ruskoline/Golden breadcrumbs
Vegetable Oil 2 tablespoons

Method:

1. Wash, peel and chop up the potatoes if using fresh and place in pan of salted water and boil until tender.

2. Drain tuna and finely chop parsley if using fresh then place tuna and parsley in a bowl and mix.

3. Remove potatoes from heat when tender and mash with the butter and milk (if required). If using pre-mashed potatoes tip them into a bowl.

4. Stir in the grated cheese then the tuna and parsley. Check seasoning then allow to cool slightly.

5. Turn tuna mixture on to a lightly floured work surface and roll into a sausage shape.

6. Place mixture into the fridge for 1 hour to chill.

7. Place the breadcrumbs into a shallow bowl like a pudding bowl.

8. Beat the egg in a bowl and season with salt and pepper then place the flour on a plate or piece of kitchen paper.

9. Remove mixture from the fridge then cut into 4 even slices to make the fishcakes.

10. Dip each fishcake in the flour, then the egg and then the breadcrumbs / ruskoline and place on a plate.

11. Heat oil in pan and fry the fishcakes for 3-4 minutes on each side until golden brown and hot all the way through. Remove from heat and drain on clean kitchen paper. Serve.

Smoked Haddock Risotto

Ingredients:

Arborio (risotto) Rice   75g (1 cup / ½ mug)
Chicken stock cubes/stock pots   1 dissolved in 450mls boiling water
Onion   ½ small fresh or 25g (1 tablespoon) frozen/fresh ready prepared diced onion
Smoked Haddock   1 fillet (skin removed)
Broccoli   fresh or frozen - 50g (2-3 florets)
Courgette   fresh - Small piece (¼)
Salt and Pepper
Vegetable Oil   15mls (1 tablespoon)

Serves 2

Method:

1. Prepare vegetables as follows if using fresh:
   - Onion - Peel and dice
   - Broccoli - Wash and cut into small florets
   - Courgette - Wash and cut into ¼ slices
2. Place broccoli and courgette into a bowl and reserve.
3. Cut fish into even-sized cubes and place in a bowl.
4. Place onion into a non-stick frying pan/pan with the oil and lightly saute (gently fry) without browning for 2-3 minutes with the lid on.
5. Add the rice to the pan and stir to coat.
6. Add the hot stock to the pan, bring to the boil and simmer for 10 minutes or until the liquid has reduced by half.
7. Add the broccoli and courgette and cook for 3-4 minutes.
8. Add the fish and cook for a further 3-4 minutes until the liquid is reduced.
9. Check seasoning and serve (maybe with a little parmesan.)

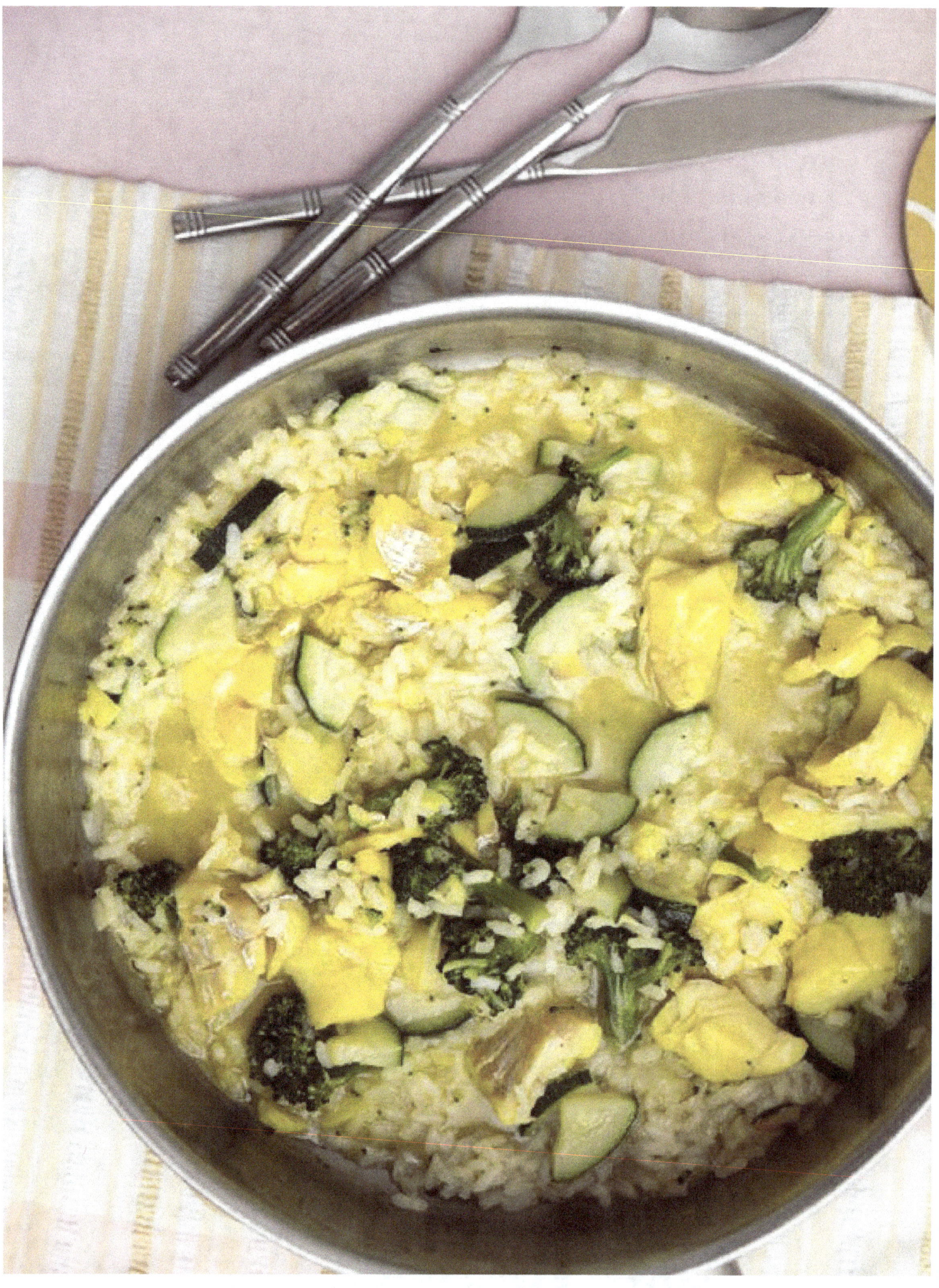

Mix and Match Pizza

PICK ONE BASE:

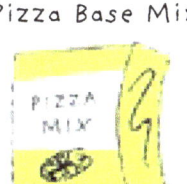
1 Packet of Pizza Base Mix

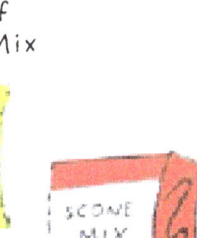
1 Packet of Scone Mix

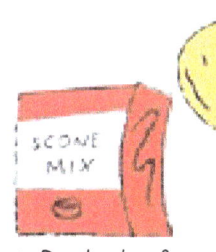
1 Large Naan Bread

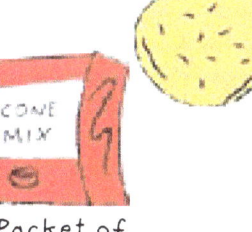
1 Pre-made pizza dough

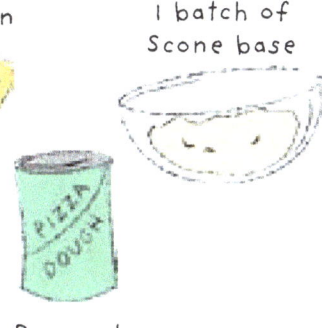
1 batch of Scone base

PICK ONE SAUCE:

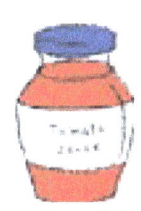
1 Jar **OR** ½ Tin Pizza sauce

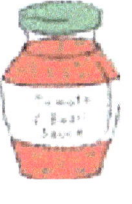
15mls (1 tablespoon) Hoisin Sauce

1 batch Tomato & Basil Sauce

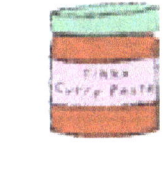
15mls (1 tablespoon) Tikka Curry Paste

30mls (2 tablespoons) Tomato Puree

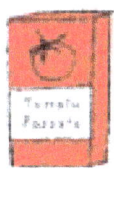
30mls (2 tablespoons) Tomato Passata

PICK A CHEESE:

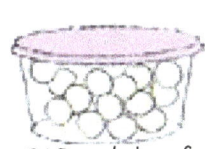
210 g tub of Mozzarella Pearls – drained

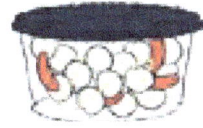
200g tub of Mozzarella Pearls and Slow Roasted Tomatoes

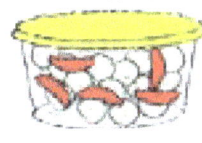
210g tub of Vine Tomatoes With Pesto Mozzarella Pearls

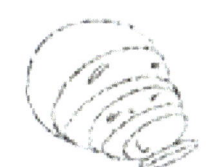
125g ball of Mozzarella – drained and sliced

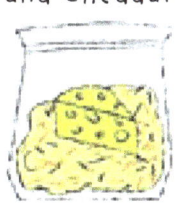
50g (2 tablespoons) Grated Mozzarella and Cheddar

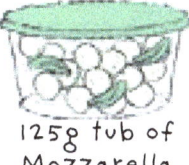
125g tub of Mozzarella Pearls with Basil

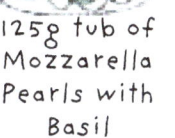
50g (2 tablespoons) Grated Chilli Cheddar

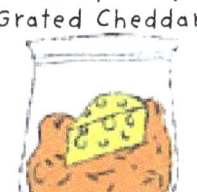
50g (2 tablespoons) Grated Cheddar

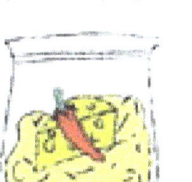
50g (2 tablespoons) Grated Mozzarella

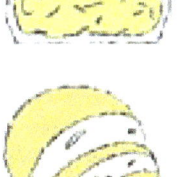
200G Smoked Mozzarella – sliced

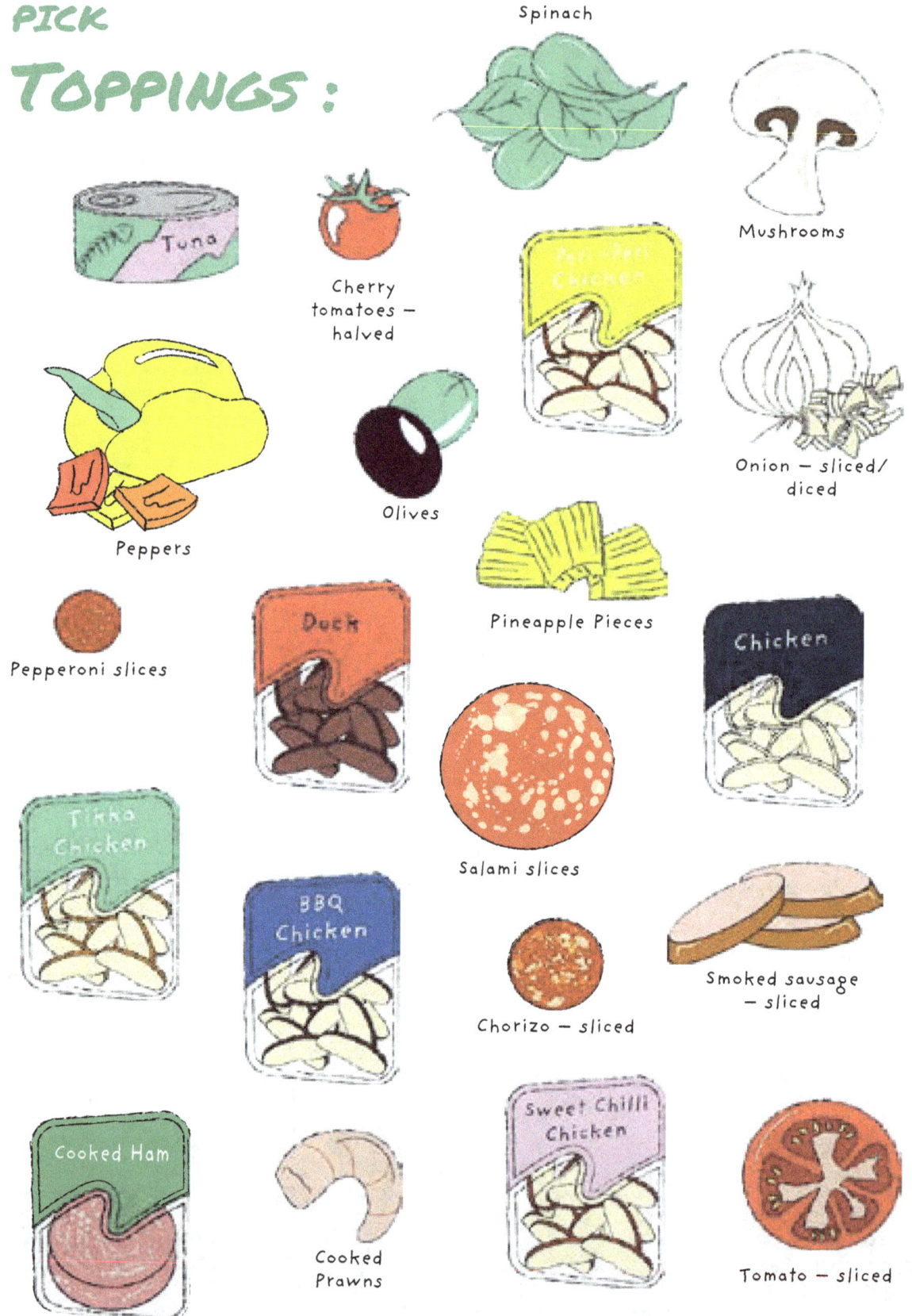

Mini Margarita Pizzas

Ingredients:

Pizza Base   1 packet pizza base mix
Pizza Topping   50mls (2 tablespoons)
Cheese   50g (2 tablespoons) grated cheddar and mozzarella
Cherry Tomatoes   2 (sliced)

Method:

1. Set oven to Gas Mark 6, 190°C
2. Place pizza base mix into large bowl and mix to a soft but not too sticky dough with the warm water as per the packet instructions.
3. Turn mixture out on to a floured surface and knead until smooth.
4. Divide the mixture into four even pieces and roll out into to four identical circles
5. Divide the topping between the four circles and spread carefully to within ½ cm of the edge.
6. Sprinkle cheese over each pizza and place the tomatoes evenly on to each of the pizzas.
7. Bake in the oven for 5-10 minutes until golden brown and base is cooked.

Calzone Pizza

Method:

1. Once you've made your pizza dough roll out to a circle.
2. Spread the sauce, cheese, and topping ingredients on to one half of the circle.
3. Dampen the edge of the half of the dough with the filing on it and fold other half to seal in filling.
4. Press down the edges with a fork to seal it.
5. Spray / brush a little oil over the top then bake in the oven for 10-15 minutes until golden.

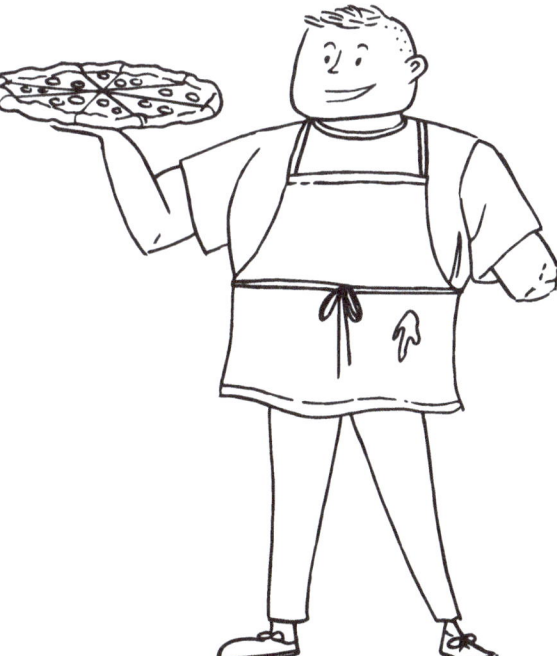

Sweet Pizzas
Method:

1. Make up a batch of pizza dough mix and roll out to a circle.
2. Heat a non-stick frying pan and place pizza base in pan and cook for 3-4 mins.
3. Turn pizza base over in the pan and place back on the heat to cook other side on a low heat.
4. Spread chocolate spread over the surface whilst the base is cooking.
5. Slice banana and place over the chocolate spread.
6. Place marshmallows over the bananas then grill until marshmallows are melted and turning golden and the chocolate spread and bananas have warmed up.
7. Serve with vanilla ice-cream.

Suggested Pizza Combos:

1.
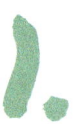 1 Pre-made pizza dough
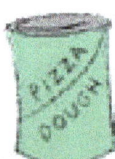 15mls (1 tablespoon) Hoisin Sauce
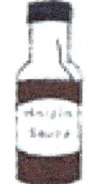 125g ball of Mozzarella – drained and sliced
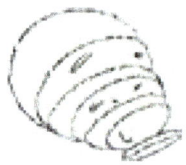 Cooked Duck

2.
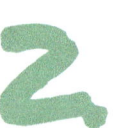 1 Large Naan Bread
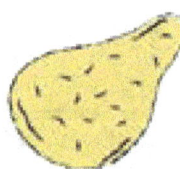 15mls (1 tablespoon) Tikka Curry Paste
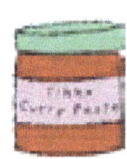 50g (2 tablespoons) Grated Mozzarella and Cheddar
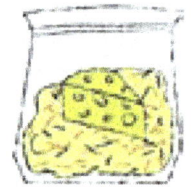 Tikka Chicken

3.
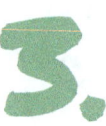 1 Packet of Pizza Base Mix
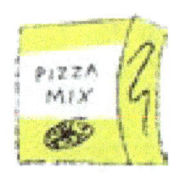 1 Jar OR ½ Tin Pizza sauce
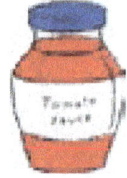 210 g tub of Mozzarella Pearls – drained
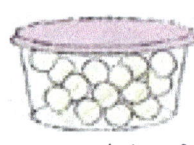 Pineapple Pieces
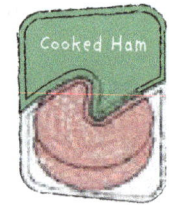 Cooked Ham

Christmas Pizzas
with the kids
Ingredients:

Mini Margarita Pizza base   1 batch (see above)
Pizza sauce   1 tablespoon

Christmas Tree
Red & Green Pepper   4 to 6 slices
Cherry tomatoes   2

Snowman
Black olives   2
Cherry tomatoes   1
Red or Green Pepper   2 slices

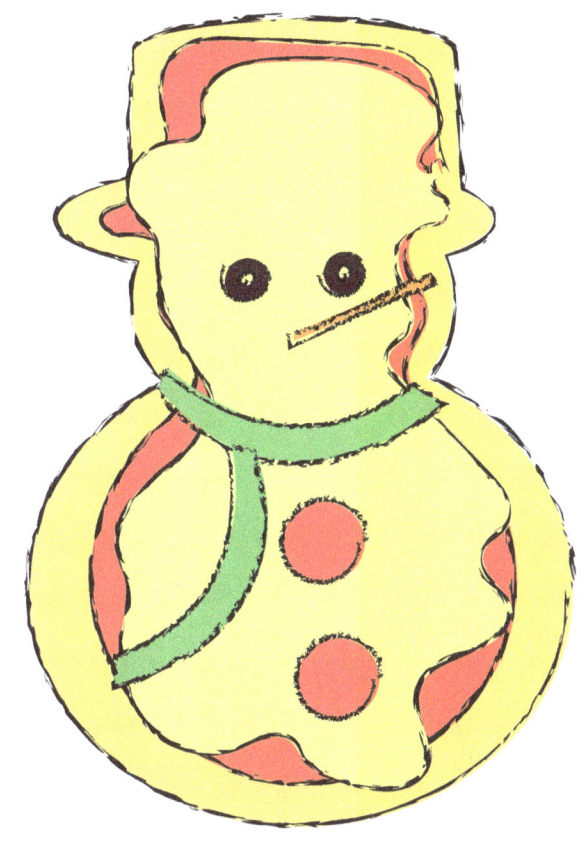

Method:

1. Set out equipment and turn oven on to Gas Mark 6, 190°C
2. Make up batch of pizza base mix.
3. Turn mixture out on to a floured surface and knead until smooth.
4. Shape the dough using the following template.
5. Mix the pizza topping and cheese together and carefully spread over the pizzas.
6. Use the decorations suggested to finish off the pizzas and bake in the oven for 8 – 10 minutes until golden brown and base is cooked.

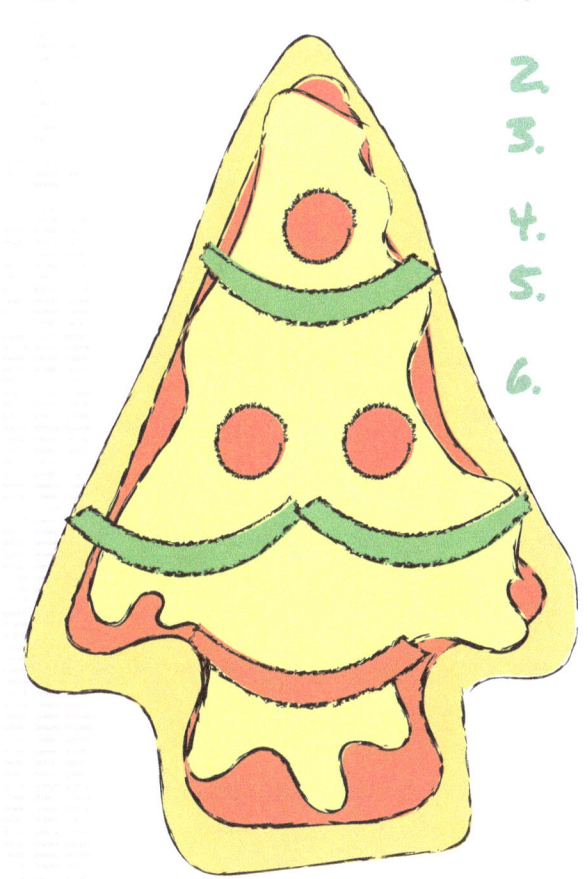

Easter Bunny Pizza
with the kids
Ingredients:

Pizza Base 1 packet pizza base mix

Decoration:
Cherry tomatoes 2
Black olives 2
Red pepper 1 slice
Pineapple 2 chunks/slices
or
Mushroom 1
Mozzarella 4 pearls / slices (optional)

Method:

1. Turn oven on to Gas Mark 6, 190°C.
2. In a bowl make up batch of pizza base mix.
3. Turn mixture out on to a floured surface and knead until smooth - this can also be done in a food processor.
4. Divide dough into four equal pieces.
5. Roll out 2 pieces of dough to give to circles and place on a baking tray.
6. Divide one of the other pieces in two and shape each piece into ears and attach to one of the circles.
7. Mix the pizza topping and cheese together and carefully spread over the pizza as per the picture.
8. Use the pineapple chunk or a slice of mushroom for the nose.
9. Slice the olives into four circles for the eyes.
10. Cut the slice of red pepper in two and use for the mouth.
11. Use the mozzarella if using to make cheeks.
12. Bake in the oven for 5-7 minutes until base is cooked and topping is golden brown.

Cheat's Lamb Curry

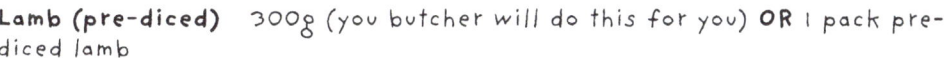

Ingredients:

Lamb (pre-diced) 300g (you butcher will do this for you) OR 1 pack pre-diced lamb
Curry Paste (Balti or Jalfrezi) 30mls (2 tablespoons)
Curry Sauce (Balti or Jalfrezi) 1 jar
Coconut Milk 1 small tin (only the milk settled on the top – NOT the coconut water) or 1 sachet coconut cream
Curry Powder (medium) 5mls (1 teaspoon) (optional)
Lamb or Beef stock cubes/stock pots 1 dissolved in 50mls (½ cup) boiling water
Long Grain Rice 150g (1 mug) OR 1 packet microwavable rice / 2 packs frozen microwaveable rice
Vegetable Oil 15mls (1 tablespoon)
Salt and Pepper

Method:

1. Place the lamb and curry paste in a bowl and stir to coat.
2. Pre-heat the oil then add the coated lamb to the pan and cook stirring all the time for 2-3 minutes.
3. Add the jar of sauce, stock pot/crumbled stock cube and stir until stock has dissolved.
4. Add the cream from the can of coconut milk (do not use the coconut water) or the sachet of coconut cream.
5. Cover with a lid and cook on a low heat for 40 minutes or transfer to a slow cooker and cook on low for approximately 5 – 6 hours.
6. Bring a pan of salted water to the boil.
7. Place rice in a sieve and rinse under the cold water tap to remove the starch then add it to the boiling water and simmer for 15 minutes until soft.
8. Drain the rice in a sieve and rinse with boiling water or prepare the microwave rice according to the instructions on the packet.
9. Taste the curry, check the seasoning and add the curry powder for a stronger flavour if desired. You can also add a dessertspoon of beef gravy granules to thicken it and enhance the flavour.

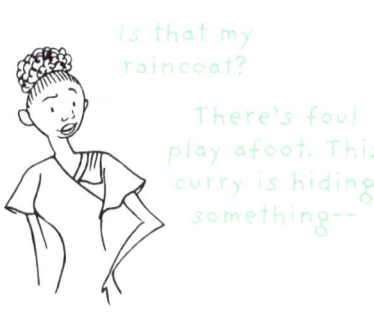

Is that my raincoat?

There's foul play afoot. This curry is hiding something--

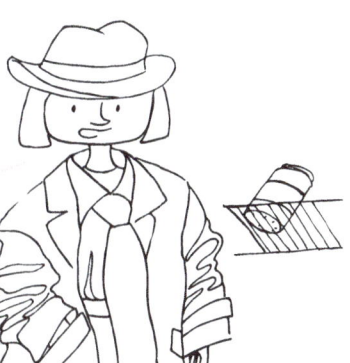

Cheat's Chicken Tikka

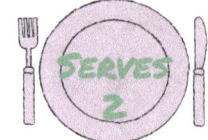

Ingredients:

Chicken Fillet (uncooked) 2 (diced) (ask a butcher to do this for you)
OR 300g pack of pre-diced chicken OR ½ pack (320g) of frozen diced uncooked chicken
Curry Paste (Tikka) 30mls (2 level tablespoons)
Coconut Milk 1 small tin (only the milk settled on the top, not the coconut water) OR 1 sachet coconut cream
Curry Powder (Tikka) 5mls (1 teaspoon) (optional)
Chicken stock cubes/stock pots 1 dissolved in 50mls (½ a cup) boiling water
Vegetable Oil 15mls (1 tablespoon)
Long Grain Rice 150g (1 mug) OR 1 packet microwave rice /2 packs frozen microwaveable rice
Salt and Pepper

Method:

1. Place the chicken and curry paste in a bowl and stir to coat.
2. Pre-heat the oil then add the coated chicken to the pan and cook stirring all the time for 2-3 minutes.
3. Add the jar of sauce, stock pot/crumbled stock cube and stir until stock has dissolved.
4. Add the cream from the can of coconut milk (do not use the coconut water) or the sachet of coconut cream.
5. Cover with a lid and cook on a low heat for 30 minutes or transfer to a slow cooker and cook on low for approximately 5 - 6 hours.
6. Bring a pan of salted water to the boil.
7. Place rice in a sieve and rinse under the cold water tap to remove the starch then add it to the boiling water and simmer for 15 minutes until soft.
8. Drain the rice in a sieve and rinse with boiling water or prepare the microwave rice according to the instructions on the packet.
9. Taste the curry, check the seasoning and add the curry powder for a stronger flavour if desired.
10. Taste the curry, check the seasoning and add the curry powder for a stronger flavour if desired. You can also add a dessertspoon of chicken gravy granules to thicken it and enhance the flavour.

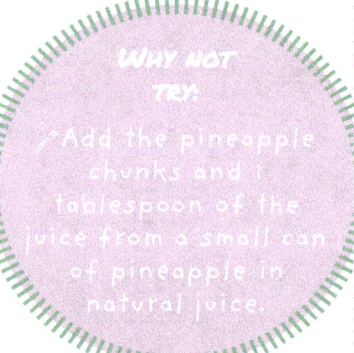

Why not try:
Add the pineapple chunks and 1 tablespoon of the juice from a small can of pineapple in natural juice.

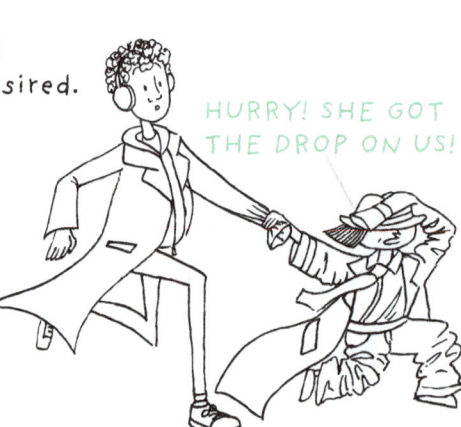

HURRY! SHE GOT THE DROP ON US!

Spicy Chicken Risotto

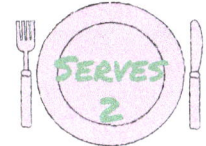

Ingredients:

Chicken Fillet (uncooked) 2 (diced) (ask a butcher to do this for you) OR 300g pack of pre-diced chicken OR ½ pack (320g) of frozen diced uncooked chicken
Arborio (risotto) Rice 150g (1 mug)
Chicken stock cubes/stock pots 1 dissolved in 450mls boiling water
Onion 1 small fresh OR 50g (2 tablespoons) frozen/fresh ready prepared diced onion
Red / Green Pepper ½ fresh or 50g (2 tablespoons) ready prepared OR frozen mixed peppers
Sweetcorn (frozen) 50g (2 tablespoons)
Curry Paste 15mls (1 tablespoon)
Vegetable or Garlic Oil 30mls (2 tablespoons)

Method:

1. Measure rice into the small bowl.
2. Peel and dice onion the onion if using fresh.
3. Wash de-seed and dice the pepper if using fresh and place in a bowl with the frozen sweetcorn.
4. Cut the chicken into cubes if using fillets.
5. Place the chicken stock cube into a measuring jug and dissolve in 250mls of boiling water.
6. Add the curry paste to the jug of stock.
7. Place the diced chicken and onion into a frying pan along with the oil and pan fry until it is starting to turn golden brown.
8. Add the rice and stock mixture to the pan.
9. Bring to the boil then simmer gently with the lid on for approximately 10 minutes until the liquid has reduced by half.
10. Add the red pepper and sweetcorn to the pan and stirring all the time allow the mixture to reduce until very little liquid is left in the pan.
11. Check taste and season if necessary with salt and pepper.
12. Transfer to serving dish.

Mozzarella and Chicken Bake

Ingredients:

Chicken Tempura Mini Chicken Fillets 300g pack
Onion 1 small fresh or 50g (2 tablespoons) frozen/fresh ready prepared diced onion
Red / Green Pepper ½ fresh or 50g (2 tablespoons) ready prepared or frozen mixed peppers
Garlic 1 clove (crushed) or 2.5mls (½ teaspoon) frozen pre-chopped/lazy garlic/garlic puree/garlic powder
Celery ½ stalk (sliced) – (optional)
Chopped Tomatoes (tinned) 1 small tin (200ml) or ½ large tin
Chicken stock cubes/stock pots/Oxo 1 dissolved in 100mls (1 cup) boiling water
Tomato Puree 15mls (1 level tablespoon)
Tomato Ketchup 5mls (1 teaspoon)
Sugar 2.5mls (½ teaspoon)
Basil (fresh or pre-frozen) 10mls (2 teaspoons) or 5mls dried (1 teaspoon)
Mozzarella Cheese 125g ball (drained)
Parmesan (grated) 1 tablespoon
Vegetable or Garlic Oil 15mls (1 tablespoon)

Serves 2

Serving suggestion:

Serve with a crispy green salad with a balsamic dressing.

Method:

1. Put oven on to Gas Mark 5, 190°C.
2. Prepare vegetables as follows for the tomato sauce if using fresh:
   - Onion – peel and finely chop
   - Celery – wash and slice
   - Red pepper – wash, de-seed and dice
   - Garlic – peel and crush
   - Basil – finely chop
3. Make up stock in jug and add chopped tomatoes, tomato puree, ketchup and sugar. Add the basil to the jug.
4. Heat oil in a frying pan and sauté (gently fry) onion, celery, pepper and garlic until soft.
5. Add contents of the jug and add a little salt and pepper.
6. Bring to the boil then reduce heat and simmer for 20 minutes until mixture thickens. Remove from heat and check seasoning.
7. For assembly, drain and slice the mozzarella.
8. Place half the tempura chicken fillets in an ovenproof dish.
9. Cover with half the tomato sauce and then half the mozzarella and parmesan cheese. Repeat this again and finish with the cheese on the top.
10. Bake uncovered for 20-30 minutes until golden brown.

Spicy Meatballs with Cheese and Chive Dip

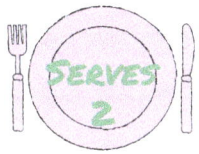

Ingredients:

Spicy Meatballs:
Minced Beef   250g fresh or frozen
Breadcrumbs (fresh)   2 tablespoons
Egg   1 (medium)
Chilli Powder   1.25mls (¼ teaspoon)
Salt   1.25mls (¼ teaspoon)
Black Pepper   pinch

Dip:
Cream Cheese   25mls (1 tablespoon)
Natural Yoghurt   25mls (1 tablespoon)
Mayonnaise   25mls (1 tablespoon)
Chives (fresh)   5mls (1 teaspoon) chopped or 1.25mls (¼ teaspoon) dried chives
Cheese (grated)   25g (1 tablespoon)

Method:

1. For the dip, place all ingredients for the dip in a clean bowl and blend using a wooden spoon or fork.

2. Place into serving dish, cover and place in the fridge until needed.

3. Place all ingredients for the meatballs into a bowl and mix with your hand or a fork.

4. Turn mixture out on to a clean board and divide into equal dessertspoonful sized portions.

5. Roll each piece into a ball using a little flour to prevent mixture sticking to hands.

6. Place on to a baking tray and bake in oven for 10 minutes until cooked all the way through.

7. Remove baking tray from the oven and place the meatballs on to kitchen paper to drain.

8. Serve either hot or cold along with the dip.

Chicken Pie

Ingredients:

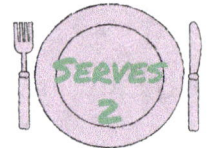

Condensed Mushroom or Chicken Soup   1 tin
Chicken stock cubes/stock pots/Oxo   1
Milk   50mls (½ cup)
Chicken Fillets Cooked   2 (sliced) or ½ bag (180g) pre-sliced cooked frozen chicken
Mushrooms   2-3 fresh or 2 tablespoons tinned or frozen sliced mushrooms (optional)
Ready Rolled Puff Pastry   1 pack (fresh) or 1 large block of puff pastry (defrosted)
Milk   1 tablespoon for glazing

Method:

1. Set the oven to Gas Mark 6, 200°C.

2. Unroll the pastry. Place the pie dish upside down on to the pastry and cut around it to make the lid for the pie (you might need to use a little flour on the work surface to stop it sticking).

3. Mark slits in the top of the pastry and cut a cross in the centre as per diagram below.

4. Place the soup, stock and milk into a pan and heat through stirring all the time to mix well and to dissolve the stock cube/pot. This will make the sauce for the pie.

5. Remove the sauce from the heat.

6. Remove the skin from the chicken if using fresh and cut into bite-sized chunks.

7. Clean and chop the mushrooms if using them.

8. Stir the cooked chicken (no need to defrost the chicken if using frozen) and mushrooms into the sauce and transfer to the pie dish.

9. Cut a few strips of the leftover pastry (approximately 2cm wide). Dampen the edge of the pie dish with a little water and stick the strips of pastry around the edge of the dish to make a border of pastry.

10. Dampen the border of pastry with milk and place the lid over the pie mix, (slit side up) attaching it to the border.

11. Seal the edges of the pastry by pressing the lid and border together with the thumb.

12. Brush the top of the pastry with milk.

13. Bake in the oven until the pastry is cooked and golden brown.

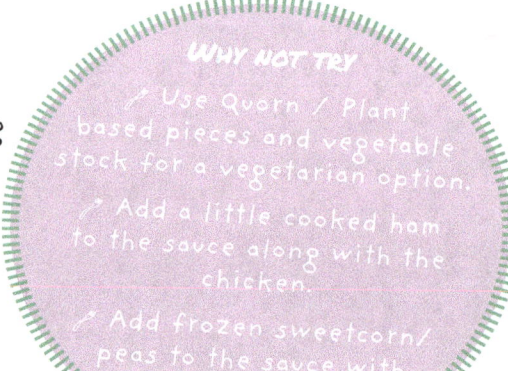

Why not try

- Use Quorn / Plant based pieces and vegetable stock for a vegetarian option.
- Add a little cooked ham to the sauce along with the chicken.
- Add frozen sweetcorn/ peas to the sauce with the chicken.

Mock Mousakka

Ingredients:

Minced Beef 250g fresh or frozen
Onion 1 small fresh or 50g (2 tablespoons) frozen/fresh ready prepared diced onion
Potatoes 2 large
Beef stock cubes/stock pots/Oxo 1 dissolved in 100mls (1 cup) boiling water
Chopped Tomatoes (tinned) 1 small tin (200ml) or ½ large tin
Mixed Herbs (dried) 1.25mls (¼ teaspoon)
Egg 1 (medium)
Natural Yogurt 1 small carton (120mls)
Milk 100mls (1 cup)
Cheese - cheddar (grated) 75g (3 tablespoons)

Serves 2

Serving Suggestions:

Serve with a crispy green salad with a balsamic dressing and some crusty garlic bread or serve with some boiled sweetcorn and peas.

Method:

1. Set oven to Gas Mark 5, 190°C.
2. Grease an ovenproof dish with either margarine or butter (try using garlic butter for added flavour).
3. Peel and finely chop the onion if using fresh.
4. Peel and finely slice the potatoes and leave to soak in cold water.
5. Brown the mince and onion in a pan and cook for 2 minutes.
6. Add the herbs, tomato and stock to the pan and cook for 1 minute.
7. Drain the sliced potatoes through a sieve then dry in a clean tea towel.
8. Place half of the sliced potatoes in the bottom of the greased ovenproof dish.
9. Put all the meat mixture on top of the potatoes and cover this with the other half of the potatoes.
10. Beat the yogurt, milk and egg together, add salt and pepper and ¾ of the cheese.
11. Pour this mixture over the meat and potatoes.
12. Sprinkle the rest of the cheese over the top.
13. Bake for 30 minutes until golden brown and the potatoes are cooked.

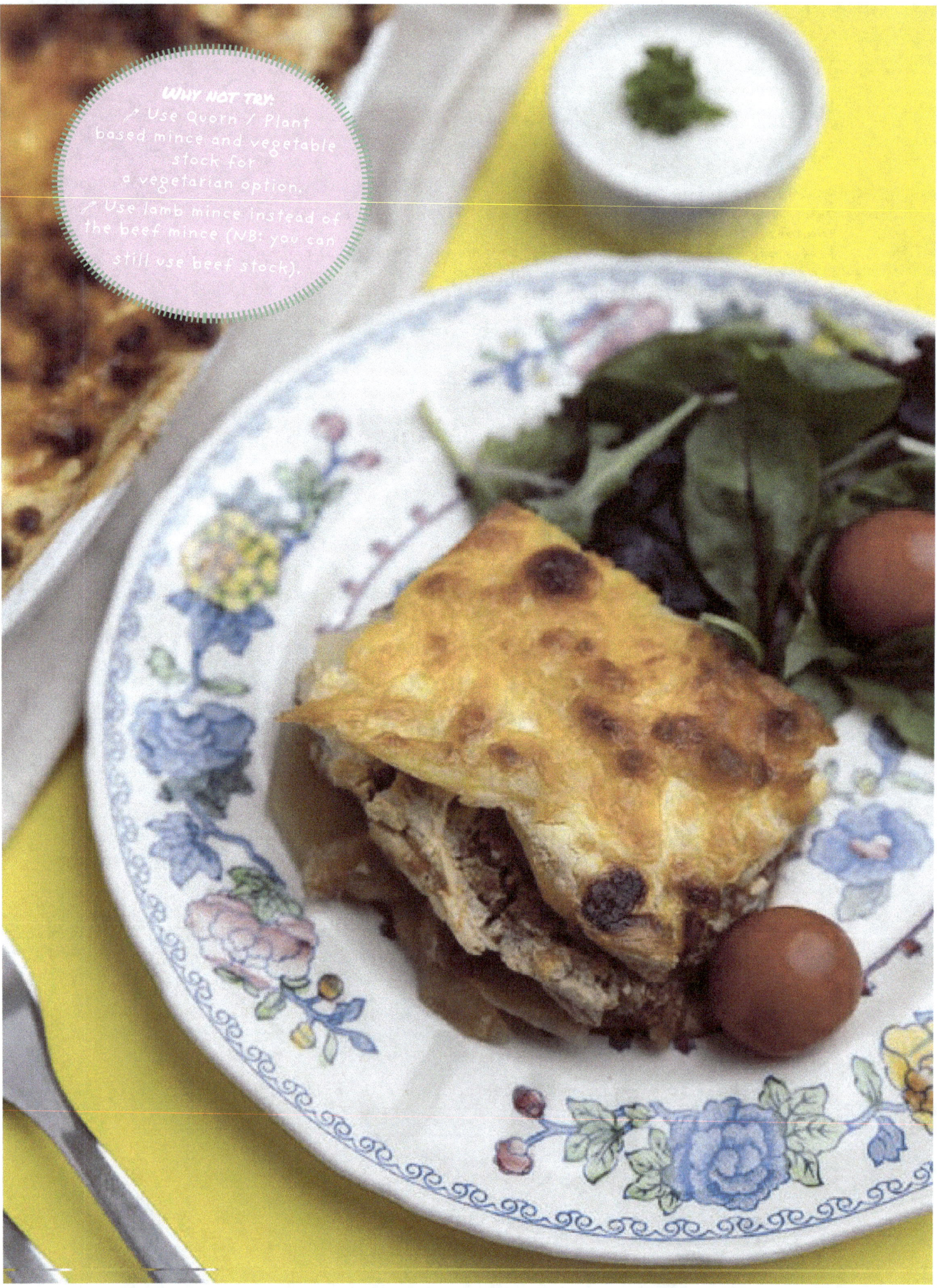

WHY NOT TRY:
- Use Quorn / Plant based mince and vegetable stock for a vegetarian option.
- Use lamb mince instead of the beef mince (NB: you can still use beef stock).

Pizza Whirls

Ingredients:

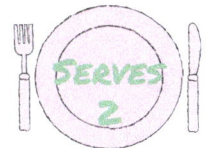

Pizza Base Mix 1 packet (145g)
Warm water to mix
Pizza Topping Mix 1 to 2 tablespoons
Cheese (grated) 50g (2 tablespoons) (cheddar, mozzarella or a mixture of both)
Mixed Herbs (dried) Pinch (optional)

Method:

1. Turn oven on to Gas Mark 6, 200°C
2. Place pizza base mix into a large bowl.
3. Mix in enough warm water as per the instructions on the packet to make a soft, but not too sticky dough.
4. Turn mixture on to a lightly floured work surface and knead until smooth.
5. Roll out dough into a long rectangle; it is important that it does not stick to the table.
6. Spread pizza topping evenly over pizza base to within 1cm of the edge.
7. Cover with the grated cheese.
8. Roll mixture up like a long swiss roll shape.
9. Cut into thin slices and lay cut side down on to a baking tray.
10. Bake in the oven for 7-10 minutes until golden brown.

Serving Suggestion: These whirls can be eaten hot or cold to reheat place in a moderate oven for 5-10 minutes.
Why not try a change: Add some finely chopped ham, drained tuna, finely chopped mushrooms or different types of cheeses such as mozzarella, blue cheese.

Vegetable Stir-fry

Ingredients:

Carrot – 1 medium fresh OR 100g (1 mug) ready prepared fresh carrot batons/frozen sliced
Onion – 1 small fresh OR 50g (2 tablespoons) frozen/fresh ready prepared diced onion
Red / Green Pepper – ½ fresh or 50g (2 tablespoons) ready prepared OR frozen mixed peppers
Courgette – fresh – Small piece (¼)
Mushrooms – 2-3 fresh OR 2 tablespoons tinned or frozen sliced mushrooms
Sweetcorn (frozen) – 50g (2 tablespoons)
Garlic – 1 clove (crushed) OR 2.5mls (½ teaspoon) frozen pre-chopped/lazy garlic/garlic puree/garlic powder
Vegetable or Garlic Oil – 30mls (2 tablespoons)
Soy Sauce – 30mls (2 tablespoons)

Serves 2

Serving Suggestions:

Serve with some crusty or garlic bread or boil some noodles or rice and stir fry with the vegetables before serving.

Method:

1. Prepare vegetables as follows if using fresh:
    - Peel and cut carrot into strips
    - Peel and slice onion
    - Wash and cut peppers into even-sized strips
    - Wash and slice the courgette
    - Wash and slice the mushrooms
    - Peel and crush the garlic

2. Place all of the vegetable into a large bowl and add the sweetcorn to the bowl.

3. Heat the oil in a frying pan, add all the vegetables and stir fry, stirring all of the time, for 2-3 minutes (vegetables should still be crisp).

    (NB: You must control the heat of your hob as the vegetables will burn if it is too hot or go soggy if it is too cold).

4. Remove pan from the heat and add the soy sauce.

5. Check for seasoning.

Why not try:
- Add cooked chicken or prawns to the vegetables when the vegetables are almost cooked and heat through until piping hot.
- Add a sachet of stir fry sauce instead of the soy sauce.
- Swap or add your vegetables – e.g. baby sweetcorn, pak choi, spring onions.

Moroccan Chicken

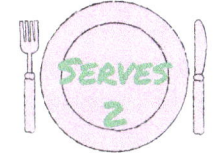

Ingredients:

Chicken Fillet (uncooked) 2 (diced) OR ½ a pack of pre-diced fresh OR frozen chicken
Ginger (ground) 5mls (1 teaspoon)
Cumin (ground) 5mls (1 teaspoon)
Paprika (ground) 5mls (1 teaspoon)
Garlic 2 cloves (crushed) OR 5mls (1 teaspoon) frozen pre-chopped/lazy garlic/garlic puree/garlic powder
Onion 1 small fresh OR 50g (2 tablespoons) frozen/fresh ready prepared diced onion
Apricots (Ready to eat dried – chopped) 50g (2 tablespoons)
Prunes (Ready to eat) 25g (1 tablespoon)
Vegetable Oil 30mls (2 tablespoons)
Cinnamon stick 1
Chopped Tomatoes (tinned) 1 small tin (200ml) OR ½ large tin
Chicken stock cubes/stock pots/Oxo 1 dissolved in 150mls (½ a mug) boiling water
Chickpeas (tinned) 1 small tin (drained)
Salt and Pepper

Method:

1. Mix the garlic with the ginger, cumin and paprika in a food bag to make the spice marinade.

2. Defrost frozen chicken or cut the fresh into even, bite-sized pieces and place in the bag with the spice marinade.

3. Coat the chicken pieces and marinade for at least 15 minutes in the fridge (leave in the fridge overnight to enhance the depth of flavour in the chicken).

4. Finely chop the onion.

5. Dice the apricots and the prunes.

6. Heat the oil in a pan and seal the chicken pieces.

7. Add the onion to the pan and sauté (lightly fry) for 2 minutes.

8. Add the apricots, prunes, cinnamon stick, tomatoes, chicken stock and chickpeas.

9. Bring to the boil, reduce the heat, cover and simmer for 20 minutes.

10. Remove the cinnamon stick and adjust the consistency and seasoning if necessary.

11. Serve in a clean, hot dish with the couscous.

Couscous

Ingredients:

Couscous (plain) 125 g (¼ of a packet)
Chicken stock cubes/stock pots 1 dissolved in 200mls (2 cups) boiling water
Coriander (fresh or frozen) 10mls (2 teaspoons) chopped OR 2.5 mls (½ teaspoon) dried

Serves 2

Method:

1. Place the couscous and coriander (if using dried) into a large bowl and stir in the hot chicken stock.

2. Cover with cling film and leave to stand for 5 minutes.

3. Finely chop the coriander (if using fresh) and reserve for garnish.

4. Remove the cling film from the couscous and using a fork stir the coriander through the couscous.

5. Taste and adjust the seasoning if necessary and serve with the Moroccan Chicken.

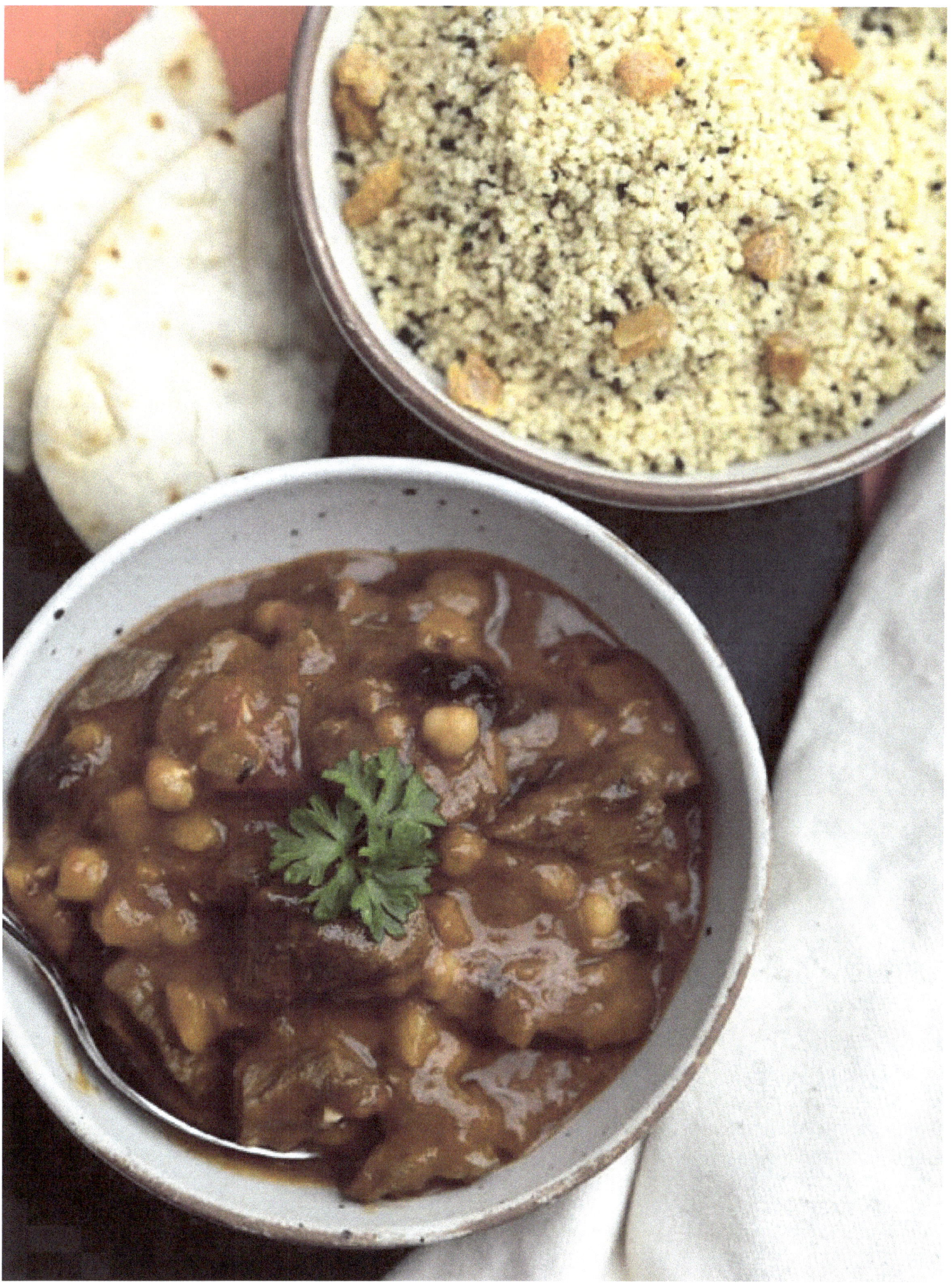

Egg Fried Rice

Ingredients:

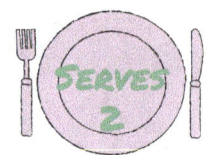

Long Grain Rice 150g (1 mug) OR 2 packets microwave rice / 4 packs frozen microwaveable rice
Vegetable Oil 30mls (2 tablespoons)
Eggs 2
Soy Sauce 30mls (2 tablespoons)
Spring Onions 2
Peas (frozen) 25g (1 tablespoon) (optional)
Salt & Pepper

Method:

1. If using microwavable rice go to step 8 of the recipe.
2. If using long grain rice, place the rice in a sieve and run under the cold water tap to remove the starch (chalky substance). When it's ready the water should run clear.
3. Place in a pan and cover with boiling water.
4. Add salt to the pan and bring to the boil over a high heat.
5. Put the lid on and turn the heat down to low. Simmer until the rice is soft.
6. Remove the pan from the heat and drain rice through a sieve.
7. Turn the rice onto a plate and spread to separate the grains.
8. Allow rice to go cold before stir frying it.
9. Wash and slice the spring onions and place in a bowl with the peas if using them.
10. Crack the eggs into a jug and beat with a fork. Add salt and pepper to the jug.
11. Heat the oil in a frying pan, add the rice and stir fry for 1 – 2 minutes to separate the grains.
12. Add the spring onions and peas to the pan and stir fry for a further minute.
13. Add the beaten egg to the pan and stir fry to cook the egg (it should look like small bits of omelette).
14. Add the soy sauce and stir to coat all the rice then serve.

Five-Spice Pork

Ingredients:

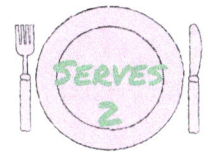

Pork Fillet (fresh) 1 trimmed of fat (butcher will do this)
Noodles (dried) 2 sections OR 1 packet fresh (cooked) noodles
Vegetable Oil 15mls (1 tablespoon)
Onion 1 small fresh OR 50g (2 tablespoons) frozen/fresh ready prepared diced onion
Garlic 1 clove (crushed) or 2.5mls (½ teaspoon) frozen pre-chopped/lazy garlic/garlic puree/garlic powder
Five-Spice Powder 5mls (1 teaspoon)
Mangetout or Sugarsnap Peas 8
Red / Green Pepper ½ fresh OR 50g (2 tablespoons) ready prepared OR frozen mixed peppers
Chicken stock cubes/stock pots/Oxo 1 dissolved in 100mls (1 cup) boiling water
Salt and Pepper
Coriander fresh leaves to garnish (optional)

Method:

1. Half fill a pan with water and put it on to boil.

2. Add the noodles to the boiling water, stir with a fork to separate then turn the heat off and leave for 4 minutes.

3. Cut the pork fillet across into thin strips (get the butcher to do this). Cover and set to one side until needed.

4. Peel and finely chop the onion if using fresh and place in a bowl.

5. Peel and crush the garlic if using fresh and put in the bowl with the onion.

6. Drain the noodles well and set aside.

7. Measure the five spice powder and place in the bowl with onion and garlic.

8. De-seed and cut the peppers into even sized strips if using fresh and cut the mangetout/sugar snap peas into even sized pieces.

9. Heat a wok or a large heavy-based frying pan until hot. Add the oil and swirl to coat the wok, then add the onion, garlic and five spice powder and stir-fry for 1 minute.

10. Add the pork strips to the wok and stir-fry for 3 minutes. Add the mangetout or sugarsnap peas and the peppers and stir-fry for a further 2 minutes. Pour in the stock, stir well and bring to the boil.

11. Add the drained noodles and stir until all the ingredients are well combined. Remove from heat and season to taste.

12. Transfer to dish and garnish with chopped coriander.

Chicken Bake

Ingredients:

Chicken Fillet (uncooked) 2 (diced) (ask a butcher to do this for you) **OR** 300g pack of pre-diced chicken **OR** ½ pack (320g) of frozen diced uncooked chicken
Sweetcorn 50g (2 tablespoons) tinned **OR** frozen sweetcorn **OR** 100g fresh broccoli cooked /100g frozen broccoli (no need to cook)
Condensed chicken soup 1 tin (295g)
Mayonnaise 50 mls (2 tablespoons)
Curry Powder 5 to 10 ml (1 to 2 teaspoons)
Crisps (plain) 2 packets (crushed)
Cheese (grated) 75g (3 tablespoon) (cheddar, mozzarella, or a mixture of both)

Method:

1. Set oven to Gas Mark 6, 200°c
2. Cut the cooked chicken into bite sized pieces.
3. Place into the bottom of an ovenproof dish.
4. Place the sweetcorn or broccoli over the top.
5. In a bowl mix the soup, mayonnaise and curry powder.
6. Pour this over the chicken and sweetcorn or broccoli and spread.
7. Mix the cheese and crisps together and sprinkle on the top.
8. Bake in the oven for 15 – 20 minutes until golden brown.

Serves 2

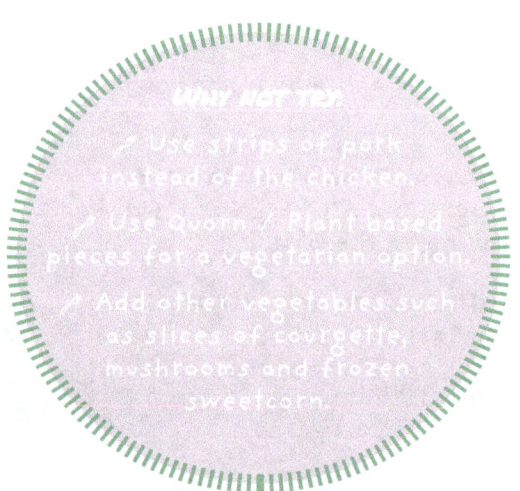

Why not try:
- Use strips of pork instead of the chicken.
- Use Quorn / Plant based pieces for a vegetarian option.
- Add other vegetables such as slices of courgette, mushrooms and frozen sweetcorn.

Chicken, Chorizo and Butternut Squash Stew

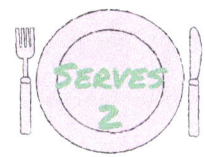

Ingredients:

Chicken Fillet (uncooked) 2 (diced) (ask a butcher to do this for you) OR 300g pack of pre-diced chicken OR ½ pack (320g) of frozen diced uncooked chicken
Chorizo (cooked and diced) ½ pack (65g) OR ¼ of a fresh cooked chorizo sausage / ¼ of a pack of frozen diced chorizo
Onion 1 small fresh OR 50g (2 tablespoons) frozen/fresh ready prepared diced onion
Butternut Squash 1 small (250g) OR ½ pack prepared fresh or frozen chunks
Garlic 2 cloves (crushed) OR 5mls (½ teaspoon) frozen pre-chopped/lazy garlic/garlic puree/garlic powder
Vegetable Oil 15mls (1 tablespoon)
Cumin (ground) 2.5mls (½ teaspoon)
Coriander fresh or pre-frozen – 2.5mls (½ teaspoon) OR 1.25mls (¼ teaspoon) dried
Tomato Puree – 15mls (1 level tablespoon)
Chopped Tomatoes (tinned) 1 large tin (400ml)
Tomato Ketchup 5mls (1 teaspoon)
Chicken stock cubes/stock pots 1 dissolved in 50mls (½ a cup) boiling water
Crème Fraiche 30ml (2 tablespoons)
Sweetcorn or Peas (or both) 75g (3 tablespoons) frozen

Method:

1. Prepare the ingredients as follows if using fresh:
   - Peel and chop the onion
   - Cut the chorizo into small chunks
   - Garlic – peel and crush
   - Cut the butternut squash into ½ across the way. Cut each half into 4. Remove the seeds and wash. Cut the skin off and then and cut into bite sized pieces.

2. Heat the oil in a pan and cook the onion and garlic stirring all the time on a low heat for 2 minutes.

3. Add the cumin and coriander and cook gently for a further minute.

4. Add the chicken and brown on each side.

5. Add the chorizo to the pan.

6. Add the butternut squash, stock cube/ stock pot, chopped tomatoes, tomato ketchup and tomato puree.

7. Bring to the boil and then simmer gently with a lid on for about 20 minutes or until the butternut squash is soft.

8. Add the peas or sweetcorn and crème fraiche to the pan and reheat to cook the vegetables.

9. Serve hot.

Chicken Jamboree

Ingredients:

Chicken Fillet (uncooked) 2 (diced) (ask a butcher to do this for you) OR 300g pack of pre-diced chicken OR ½ pack (320g) of frozen diced uncooked chicken
Chopped Tomatoes (tinned) 1 large tin (400ml)
Apricots (Ready to eat dried - chopped) 75g (3 tablespoons)
Onion 1 small fresh or 50g (2 tablespoons) frozen/fresh ready prepared diced onion
Brown Sugar 10ml (2 teaspoons)
Malt Vinegar 50mls (2 tablespoons)
Turmeric (ground) 5mls (1 teaspoon)
Ginger (ground) 5mls (1 teaspoon)
Garlic 1 clove (crushed) OR 2.5mls (½ teaspoon) frozen pre-chopped/lazy garlic/garlic puree/garlic powder
Chicken stock cubes/stock pots 1 dissolved in 50mls (½ a cup) boiling water
Vegetable Oil 15mls (1 tablespoon)
Salt and Pepper

Serves 2

Serving Suggestion:

Serve with cooked rice or Couscous

Method:

1. Prepare the ingredients as follows if using fresh:
   - Onion - Peel and chop
   - Cut the chorizo into small chunks
   - Garlic — peel and crush
2. Heat the oil in a pan. Add the chicken and stir until it is brown all over.
3. Add the turmeric, ginger and garlic and gently cook for 1 minute, stirring to coat the chicken in the spices.
4. Add the tomatoes, brown sugar, vinegar and the stock pot/cube.
5. Bring to the boil and then gently simmer with a lid on for 10 minutes.
6. Add the apricots and simmer for a further 10 minutes.

Chicken and Mango Curry

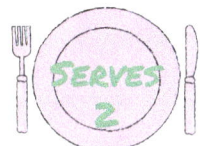

Ingredients:

Onion   1 small fresh or 50g (2 tablespoons) frozen/fresh ready prepared diced onion
Chicken Fillet (cooked)   2 (diced) OR 360g of fresh pre-diced cooked chicken / 1 pack (340g) of frozen diced cooked chicken
Garlic   2 cloves (crushed) OR 5mls (1 teaspoon) frozen pre-chopped/lazy garlic/garlic puree/garlic powder
Chicken stock cubes/stock pots   1 dissolved in 50mls (½ a cup) boiling water
Ginger (ground)   2.5mls (½ teaspoon) or 1.25mls (¼ teaspoon) Very Lazy chopped ginger
Curry Paste   10mls (2 teaspoons)
Tomato Puree   10mls (2 teaspoons)
Mango (fresh)   250g or ½ bag prepared frozen mango pieces
Crème Fraiche   30ml (2 tablespoons)
Vegetable Oil   15mls (1 tablespoon)

Method:

1. Prepare the following ingredients if using fresh:
   - Onion – Peel and chop
   - Garlic – peel and crush
   - Mango – peel and dice (see tips)
   - Cut the chicken into bite sized pieces (using a scissors is easier)

2. Heat the oil in a pan. Add the chicken and stir until it is brown all over.

3. Add the onion, garlic, curry paste, tomato puree and ginger and cook for 2 minutes.

4. Add the chicken stock.

5. Bring to the boil and simmer with a lid on for 10 minutes.

6. Add the mango and cook for a further 3 minutes.

7. Add the crème fraiche and heat through.

Beef and Sweet Potato Casserole

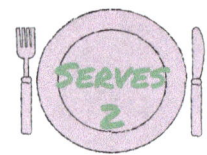

Ingredients:

Diced Beef (lean) 400g (ask your butcher to do this for you) OR 1 pack fresh lean diced beef / frozen casserole beef
Onion 1 small fresh OR 50g (2 tablespoons) frozen/fresh ready prepared diced onion
Leek 1 small OR 100g (1 cup) frozen sliced leek
Carrot 1 medium OR 100g (1 cup) prepared or frozen carrot
Butternut Squash 1 small (250g) OR ½ pack prepared fresh OR frozen chunks
Plain Flour 15ml (1 tablespoon)
Allspice (ground) 2.5mls (½ teaspoon)
Tomato Puree 15mls (1 level tablespoon)
Red Wine 100ml (1 cup)
Beef stock cubes/stock pots/Oxo 1 dissolved in 150mls (1 mug) boiling water
Chopped Tomatoes (tinned) 1 small tin (200ml) OR ½ large tin
Sweet Potatoes 200g fresh / ready prepared or frozen
Vegetable Oil 10mls (2 teaspoons)

Method:

1. Prepare the ingredients as follows if using fresh:
   - Onion — Peel and chop
   - Leek - wash, slice in half and rewash. Cut across into 1cm pieces
   - Carrots - wash, peel and cut into 1cm pieces
   - Butternut Squash — wash, peel and cut into 2 cm pieces

2. Place mince into a pan and brown on a high heat stirring all the time to break down the granules of mince. Stir in the flour and the allspice and mix.

3. Add the onion, leek, carrots and butternut squash. Gently cook for 5 minutes, stirring continuously.

4. Stir in the tomato puree, red wine, beef stock and passata or chopped tomatoes.

5. Bring to the boil and simmer gently with the lid on for 45 – 60 minutes – check to see the meat is tender.

6. Put the oven on to Gas mark 6, 200°C.

7. Wash, peel and thinly slice or cube the sweet potatoes if using fresh.

8. Check the seasoning and place the meat in a casserole dish and top with the sweet potato.

9. Spray the sweet potatoes with spray oil or brush with oil and cover with tin foil.

10. Cook in the oven for 30 minutes, remove foil and cook for a further 15 minutes until the sweet potato has browned and the beef is tender.

Beef with Apricots

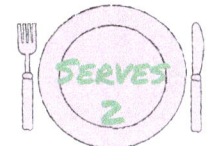

Ingredients:

Diced Beef (lean) 400g (ask your butcher to do this for you) OR 1 pack fresh lean diced beef / frozen casserole beef
Onion 1 large fresh OR 100g (4 tablespoons) frozen / fresh ready prepared diced onion
Garlic 2 cloves (crushed) OR 5mls (1 teaspoon) frozen pre-chopped / lazy garlic / garlic puree / garlic powder
Apricots (Ready to eat dried – chopped) 100g (1 cup)
Beef stock cubes/stock pots/Oxo 1 dissolved in 100mls (1 cup) boiling water
Chopped Tomatoes (tinned) 1 large tin (400ml)
Vegetable Oil 10mls (2 teaspoons)

Serving Suggestion:

Serve with some Couscous or boiled potatoes and boiled vegetables such as peas/green beans on the side.

Method:

1. Prepare the ingredients as follows if using fresh:
   - Onion – Peel and chop
   - Garlic – Peel and crush

2. Place the meat into a pan with the oil and brown on a high heat stirring all the time.

3. Add the onions and garlic and cook for about 4 minutes stirring all the time.

4. Add the tomatoes, apricots, and stock.

5. Bring to the boil and then gently simmer with the lid on for about 1 hour or until the beef is tender, stirring occasionally.

6. Check seasoning and serve.

> **Cook's Tip:**
> The whole dish could be cooked in the oven. After Step 4 place mixture in a casserole dish, cover with tinfoil and cook for 1 hour at Gas mark 6, 190°C, for 1 hour until beef is tender.

Cottage Pie with Sweet Potato Topping

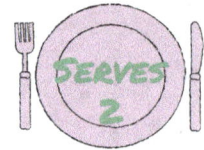

Ingredients:

Minced Beef — 250g fresh or frozen
Onion — 1 small fresh or 50g (2 tablespoons) frozen/fresh ready prepared diced onion
Garlic — 1 clove (crushed) or 2.5mls (½ teaspoon) frozen pre-chopped/lazy garlic/garlic puree/garlic powder
Carrot — 1 medium or 100g (1 cup) fresh carrot batons / frozen sliced carrots
Chopped Tomatoes (tinned) — 1 small tin (200ml) or ½ large tin
Worcestershire sauce — 10mls (2 teaspoons)
Tomato Puree — 10mls (2 teaspoons)
Beef stock cubes/stock pots/Oxo — 1 dissolved in 150mls (1 mug) boiling water
Frozen Peas — 75g (3 tablespoons)
Sweet Potato — 400g ready prepared mashed

Method:

1. Prepare the ingredients as follows if using fresh:
   - Onion — Peel and chop
   - Carrot — Wash, peel and slice
   - Garlic — Peel and crush
2. Place mince into a pan and brown on a high heat stirring all the time to break down the granules of mince.
3. Add the onion, carrots and garlic and cook for a further minute.
4. Add the tomatoes, tomato puree, Worcestershire sauce and the stock.
5. Bring to the boil and then gently simmer with the lid on for 10-15 minutes.
6. Add the peas and mix.
7. Remove from the heat.
8. Put the oven on to Gas mark 6, 190°C.
9. Place the mince mixture in a pie dish or casserole.
10. Spoon the ready prepared sweet potato over the top spread out carefully with a knife and use a fork to mark lines.
11. Bake for 20 minutes until browned.

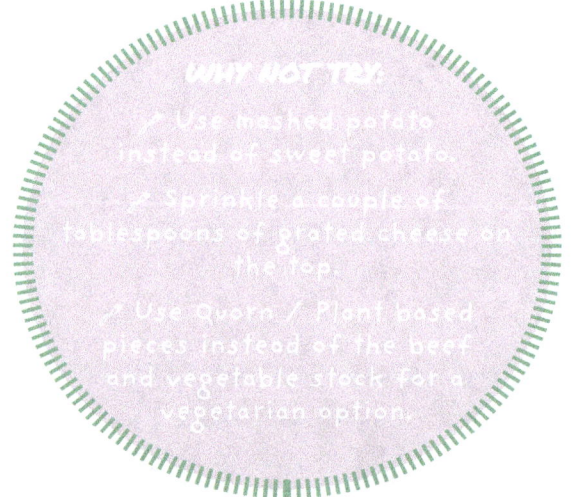

Why not try:
- Use mashed potato instead of sweet potato.
- Sprinkle a couple of tablespoons of grated cheese on the top.
- Use Quorn / Plant based pieces instead of the beef and vegetable stock for a vegetarian option.

Mediterranean Pork Casserole

Ingredients:

Pork (lean and diced)   250g (your butcher will do this for you) OR ½ a 500g pack of diced pork
Onion   1 small fresh OR 50g (2 tablespoons) frozen/fresh ready prepared diced onion
Garlic   1 clove (crushed) OR 2.5mls (½ teaspoon) frozen pre-chopped/lazy garlic/garlic puree/garlic powder
Red / Green Pepper   1 fresh OR 100g (4 tablespoons) ready prepared OR frozen mixed peppers
Chopped Tomatoes (tinned)   1 large tin (400ml)
Mushrooms   2-3 fresh or 2 tablespoons tinned OR frozen sliced mushrooms
Vegetable Oil   15ml (1 tablespoon)
Cornflour   10mls (2 teaspoons)
Smoked Paprika   5ml (1 teaspoon)
Thyme (dried)   1.25mls (¼ teaspoon)
Salt and Pepper

Serves 2

Method:

1. Prepare the ingredients as follows if using fresh:
   - Onion — Peel and chop
   - Pepper — Wash, deseed and slice
   - Garlic — Peel and crush
   - Mushrooms — Wash and slice
   - Cut the pork into bite sized pieces using a kitchen scissors

2. Heat the oil in a pan. Add the pork and stir until it is brown all over.

3. Add the onion, garlic and gently sauté for about 2 minutes.

4. Add the cornflour, smoked paprika and thyme and mix well.

5. Add the tomatoes, peppers and mushrooms.

6. Bring to the boil and either:

   Cover the pan and simmer for about 25 minutes until the pork is tender, stirring occasionally

   OR

7. Place in a casserole dish, cover with tin foil and cook at gas mark 5, 190°C fan oven for about 30 - 40 minutes until the pork is tender.

8. Taste for seasoning and add salt and pepper if required.

Pork Medallions with Creamy Mustard Sauce

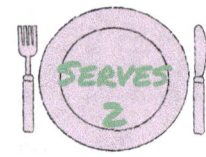

Ingredients:

Pork Medallions 6 small **OR** a 300g pack of pork fillet medallions
Red Onion 1 medium fresh **OR** 75g (3 tablespoons) frozen / fresh ready prepared diced onion
Wholegrain Mustard 30ml (2 tablespoons) – more can be added to taste
Crème Fraiche 200g (1 tub)
Vegetable Oil 15ml (1 tablespoon)
Salt and Pepper

Serving Suggestion:

Serve with some mashed / baby new potatoes or Couscous.

Method:

1. Peel and cut the red onion into wedges, slices or chopped.
2. Heat the oil in a non-stick griddle or frying pan.
3. Fry the onion gently in the oil until softened then add the medallions and fry for about 7-10 minutes, turning frequently, until the meat is thoroughly cooked – check by cutting into the centre.
4. Mix the mustard and the crème fraiche together and add to the pan Heat through then serve.

Why not try:
- Add some sliced mushrooms and cook with the pork.
- Use Quorn / Plant based pieces/medallions for a vegetarian option

Cook's Tip:
- If pork medallions are not available use thinly cut pork loin cutlets.
- This dish can also be made using chicken mini fillets.

Sausage Stew

Ingredients:

Pork Sausages 6
Onion 1 small fresh OR 50g (2 tablespoons) frozen/fresh ready prepared diced onion
Carrot 1 medium OR 100g (1 cup) fresh carrot batons / frozen sliced carrots
Celery 1 small stick (optional)
Mixed Herbs 2.5mls (½ teaspoon)
Garlic 1 clove (crushed) OR 2.5mls (½ teaspoon) frozen pre-chopped/lazy garlic/garlic puree/garlic powder
Chopped Tomatoes (tinned) 1 small tin (200ml) OR ½ large tin
Worcestershire Sauce 15ml
Tomato Ketchup 30ml (2 tablespoons)
Vegetable stock cubes/stock pots 1 dissolved in 150mls (1 mug) boiling water
Kidney Beans (tinned) 1 small tin (200ml) OR ½ large tin
Cornflour 5ml blended with 15ml water
Vegetable Oil 15ml (1 tablespoon)
Salt and Pepper

Method:

1. Prepare ingredients:
   - Peel and chop the onion
   - Wash, peel and dice the carrot
   - Wash the celery and slice thinly
   - Drain and rinse the kidney beans
   - Blend the cornflour and water together

2. Heat the oil in a frying pan and brown the sausages all over.

3. Add the onion, carrot and celery (if using) and cook about 5 minutes, stirring frequently.

4. Add the tomatoes, mixed herbs, tomato ketchup, Worcestershire sauce and stock.

5. Bring to the boil and simmer 15 minutes with a lid on or use a piece of tinfoil to form a lid.

6. Add the kidney beans. Simmer for 5 minutes, stirring frequently.

7. Add the cornflour and simmer 2 minutes.

Cook's Tip:

After step 4 of the recipe, all the ingredients could be put into a casserole and cooked in the oven Gas Mark 5, 190°C for 30 minutes.

Mixed Bean Goulash

Ingredients:

Kidney Beans (tinned) 1 small tin (200g) **OR** ½ large tin
Baked Beans (tinned) 1 small tin (200g) **OR** ½ large tin
Chopped Tomatoes (tinned) 1 small tin (200ml) **OR** ½ large tin
Onion 1 small fresh **OR** 50g (2 tablespoons) frozen/fresh ready prepared diced onion
Garlic 1 clove (crushed) **OR** 2.5mls (½ teaspoon) frozen pre-chopped/lazy garlic/garlic puree/garlic powder
Vegetable stock cubes/stock pots 1 dissolved in 150mls (1 mug) boiling water
Vegetable Oil 15ml (1 tablespoon)
Paprika 5mls (1 teaspoon)
Sugar 2.5mls (½ teaspoon)
Salt and Pepper

Serves 2

Serving Suggestions:

Serve with some boiled rice or in a pitta bread or tortilla.

Method:

1. Prepare ingredients as follows:
   - Peel and chop the onion
   - Peel and crush the garlic

2. Drain and rinse the kidney bean by putting them in a sieve and running cold water through.

3. Heat the oil in a pan and gently sauté the onion, garlic and paprika until the onion is soft.

4. Add the tomatoes, stock pot / crumbled up stock cube, baked beans and kidney beans.

5. Bring to the boil and simmer, stirring gently, for about 15 minutes until thickened and glossy.

6. Taste for seasoning and serve.

Fish Burgers with Tartare Sauce

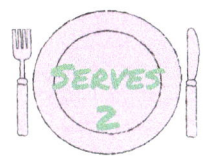

Ingredients:

Burgers:
White Fish   250g (1 large fillet)
Bread   1 slice
Egg   1 (medium)
Lime   ½ (zest and juice)
Garlic   1 clove (crushed) OR 2.5mls (½ teaspoon) frozen pre-chopped/lazy garlic/garlic puree/garlic powder
Coriander   fresh or pre-frozen - 10mls (1 dessertspoon) OR 5mls (1 teaspoon) dried
Soy Sauce   10mls (2 teaspoons)
Salt and Pepper
Vegetable Oil   30mls (2 tablespoon)

For the coating:
Natural/Panko Breadcrumbs   1 cup (½ mug) OR Ruskoline/Golden breadcrumbs
Black Sesame Seeds   5mls (1 teaspoon) (optional)

A small jar of tartare sauce can be used, if you would like to make your own use the ingredients below:

Tartare Sauce:
Mayonnaise   200mls
Dijon Mustard   2.5mls (½ teaspoon)
Capers   50g (2 tablespoons)
Gherkins   50g (2 tablespoons)
Coriander   fresh or pre-frozen - 10mls (2 teaspoons) OR 2.5mls (½ teaspoon) dried
Chilli fresh (green)   2.5mls (½ teaspoon) deseeded and roughly chopped OR ½ teaspoon pre-chopped frozen chilli
Garlic   1 small clove (crushed) OR 1.25mls (¼ teaspoon) frozen pre-chopped/lazy garlic/garlic puree/garlic powder
Lime   ½ (zest and juice)
Sugar   Pinch
Salt   Pinch

For serving:
Burger Buns   2
Lettuce   Iceberg or Little Gem - Some shredded

Serving Suggestions:

Serve with tomato salsa (see recipe) and/or a crisp green salad

Method:

1. Place all the ingredients for the burger into food processor and mix together and season.
2. Divide mixture into 2 large or 4 small patties and place on piece of foil on a baking tray.
3. Place in the freezer for 10 minutes to firm up.
4. Mix the breadcrumbs and sesame seeds (if using) for the coating in a bowl.
5. Remove the burgers from the freezer and coat with the breadcrumb and sesame seed mix.
6. Heat the oil in a frying pan and fry the burgers for 2 minutes on each side until the breadcrumbs are golden then place back on to the baking tray.
7. Bake in the oven for a further 15 – 20 minutes until they are cooked through.

Tartare Sauce:

8. Place all the ingredients into the food processor and mix well. Then place into a clean bowl, cover, and store in the fridge for up to 2 weeks.

To assemble:

9. Split the burger buns through the middle and toast each half under the grill or in the oven.
10. Spoon some tartare sauce on the bottom half of the bun and add a small bunch of shredded lettuce.
11. Place a burger on top and replace the lid.

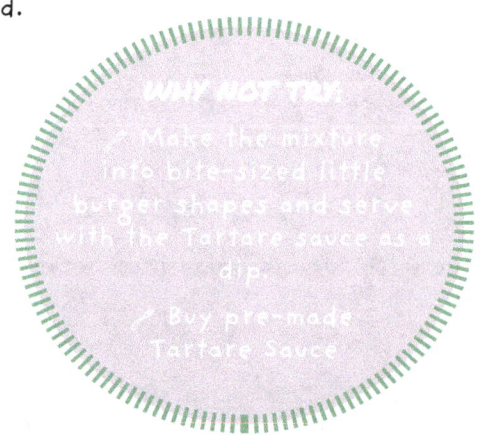

WHY NOT TRY:
- Make the mixture into bite-sized little burger shapes and serve with the Tartare sauce as a dip.
- Buy pre-made Tartare Sauce

PASTA

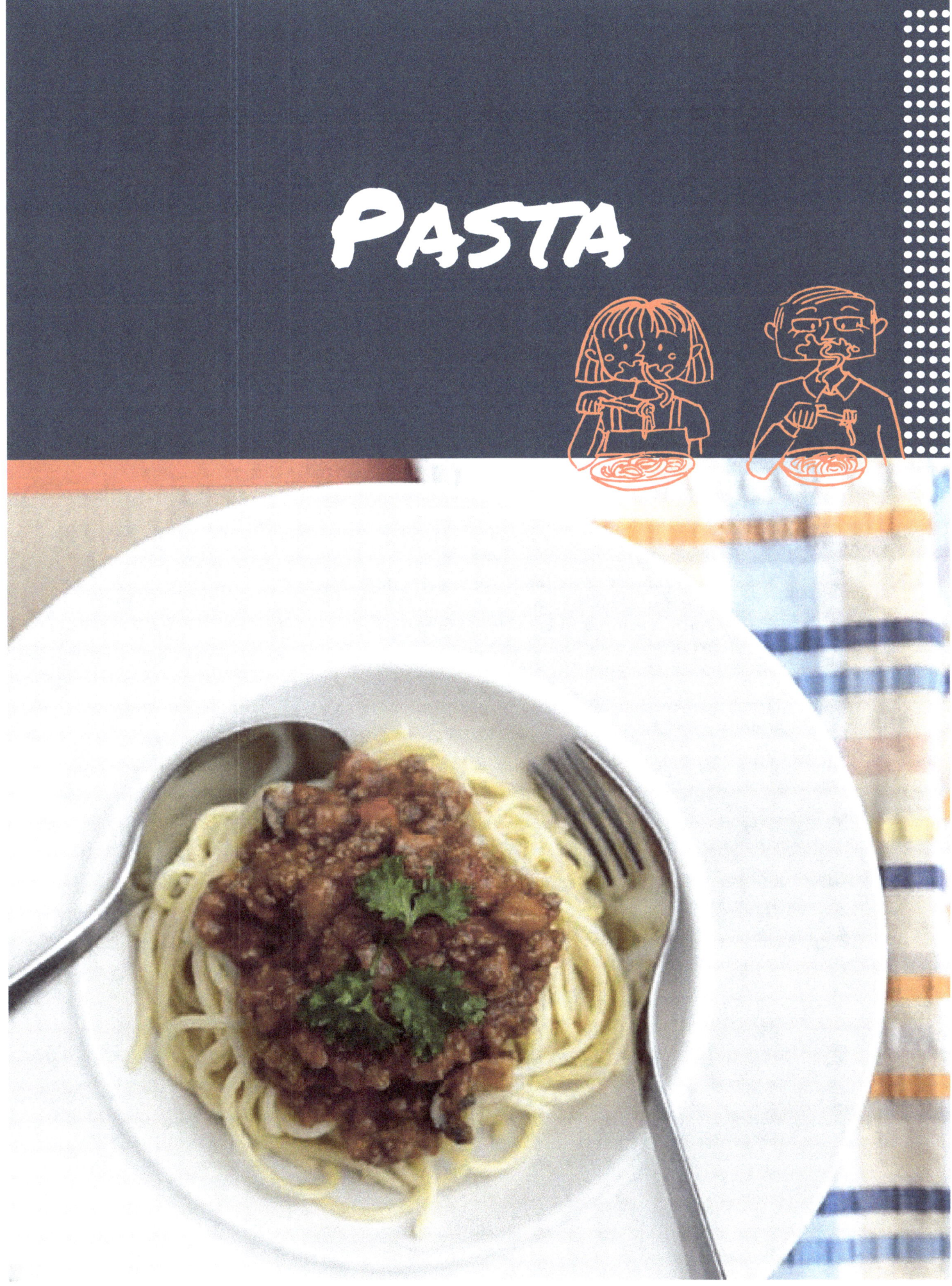

Spaghetti Bolognese

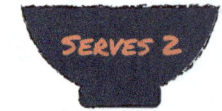

Ingredients:

Onion • 1 small fresh **OR** 50g (2 tablespoons) frozen/fresh ready prepared diced onion
Red / Green Pepper • ½ fresh **OR** 50g (2 tablespoons) ready prepared or frozen mixed peppers
Celery • 1 stalk (sliced) – (optional)
Lardons • 1 small pack (unsmoked) **OR** 1-2 rasher unsmoked back bacon (chopped)
Minced Beef • 250g fresh **OR** frozen
Tomato Puree • 15mls (1 level tablespoon)
Chopped Tomatoes (tinned) • 1 small tin (200ml) **OR** ½ large tin
Mushrooms • 2-3 fresh or 2 tablespoons tinned **OR** frozen sliced mushrooms (optional)
Mixed Herbs (dried) • 2.5mls (½ teaspoon)
Garlic • 1 clove (crushed) **OR** 2.5mls (½ teaspoon) frozen pre-chopped/lazy garlic/garlic puree/garlic powder
Beef stock cubes/stock pots/Oxo • 1 dissolved in 150mls (½ a mug) boiling water
Tomato Ketchup • 5mls (1 teaspoon)
Sugar • Pinch
Spaghetti • 150g

Method:

1. Prepare ingredients as follows if using fresh:
   - Peel and chop the onion
   - Wash, deseed and chop the pepper
   - Wash and chop the celery
   - Wash and slice mushrooms

2. Trim bacon and cut into small even sized pieces using scissors, if not using lardons.

3. Make up stock in a jug. Add tinned tomatoes, tomato puree, mixed herbs, garlic, sugar and tomato sauce to the jug.

4. Place mince in a pan and cook on a high heat, stirring all the time until the mince has broken up and turned brown.

5. Add the bacon, onion, peppers and celery to the pan and cook for a further two minutes.

6. Add the rest of the ingredients from the jug along with the mushrooms and bring to simmering point. Add a little salt and pepper to the pan.

7. Simmer with the lid on for 20 minutes until mince is cooked. Season to taste.

8. Half fill another pan with water, add salt and bring to the boil. Measure out spaghetti and break in half. Add spaghetti and boil for 10-15 minutes.

9. Make a nest in the spaghetti and spoon the bolognaise sauce carefully into the centre and serve.

Macaroni Cheese

Ingredients:

- Macaroni · 100g (1 cup)
- Plain Flour · 25g (1 tablespoon)
- Margarine · 25g (1 tablespoon)
- Milk · 300mls (2 mugs)
- Cheese (grated) · 75g (3 tablespoons)
- Tomato · 1
- Salt and Pepper

Method:

1. Half fill a pan with cold water, add ½ teaspoon salt and bring to the boil.
2. Add pasta to the boiling water and simmer for 10-12 minutes until soft.
3. Measure milk, flour, and margarine into a measuring jug and blend with a fork to breakdown flour.
4. Pour contents of jug into a pan.
5. Slowly bring mixture to the boil, stirring all the time and boil for 1-2 minutes.
6. Remove sauce from the heat, add 2/3 of the grated cheese and stir until it melts. (Do not return pan to the heat as the cheese will separate).
7. Drain pasta into a sieve.
8. Stir the pasta into the cheese sauce and season with salt and pepper.
9. Turn mixture into an ovenproof dish.
10. Sprinkle the rest of the cheese over the top.
11. Slice tomato on a chopping board then place on top of the cheese.
12. Place in a hot oven or grill to brown.

Why not try: Add some drained tuna to the sauce before placing it in the ovenproof dish to make it a tuna pasta bake or try adding some cooked ham or chicken.

Chicken Supreme

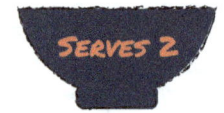

Ingredients:

Plain Flour • 25g (1 tablespoon)
Margarine • 25g (1 tablespoon)
Milk • 150mls (1mug)
Chicken stock cubes/stock pots • 1 dissolved in 150mls (½ a mug) boiling water
Onion • ½ small fresh or 25g (1 tablespoon) frozen/fresh ready prepared diced onion
Red / Green Pepper • ½ fresh or 50g (2 tablespoons) ready prepared or frozen mixed peppers
Chicken Fillet (uncooked) • 1 (thinly sliced) or 100g pre-diced fresh or frozen (defrosted) chicken
Vegetable or Garlic Oil • 15mls (1 tablespoon)
Peas (frozen) • 25g (1 tablespoon)
Sweetcorn (frozen) • 25g (1 tablespoon)
Pasta Twists or Shells • 100g (1 mug) or Long Grain Rice - 150g (1 mug) or 2 packets microwave rice / 4 packs frozen microwaveable rice

Method:

1. Half fill a pan with cold water, add ½ teaspoon salt and bring to the boil.
2. Add pasta / rice to the boiling water and simmer for 10-12 minutes until soft. Alternatively prepare the microwave rice according to the instructions on the packet.
3. Make up stock in jug and add milk to jug.
4. Add the flour and margarine to the measuring jug and stir with a fork to breakdown the flour.
5. Pour contents of jug into a pan. Slowly bring mixture to the boil, stirring all the time and boil for 1-2 minutes. Remove from heat and check the seasoning.
6. Cover pan with a damp piece of kitchen paper to prevent a skin forming.
7. Peel, wash and dice onion and pepper if using fresh.
8. Cut the chicken into thin strips.
9. Heat the oil in a frying pan and fry the chicken, onion and pepper for 5 minutes. Add the sweetcorn and peas to the pan and cook for a further 5 minutes.
10. Check that the chicken is cooked all the way through.
11. Pour the chicken and vegetable mix into the pan of sauce.
12. Drain the pasta or rice and place into an ovenproof dish.
13. Pour the chicken mixture into centre of pasta and serve.

Pasta Potage

Serves 2

Ingredients:

Pasta Twists/Shells/Penne • 200g (2 mugs)
Tomato Soup • 1 tin (400g)
Bacon • 2 rashers
Cheese (grated) • 25g (1 tablespoon) (cheddar, mozzarella or a mixture of both)

Serving suggestion:

Serve with some crusty, garlic or flat bread.

Method:

1. Put pan of salted water on to boil.
2. Put grill on to pre-heat.
3. Add pasta to pan of water and boil until soft.
4. Grill or microwave the bacon then cut up into small pieces.
5. Drain pasta through a sieve and then put it back into the pan.
6. Add the soup and the bacon to the pan.
7. Stirring all the time heat the soup through.
8. Transfer mixture to an ovenproof dish.
9. Sprinkle the grated cheese over the top and either grill or bake the dish to melt the cheese.

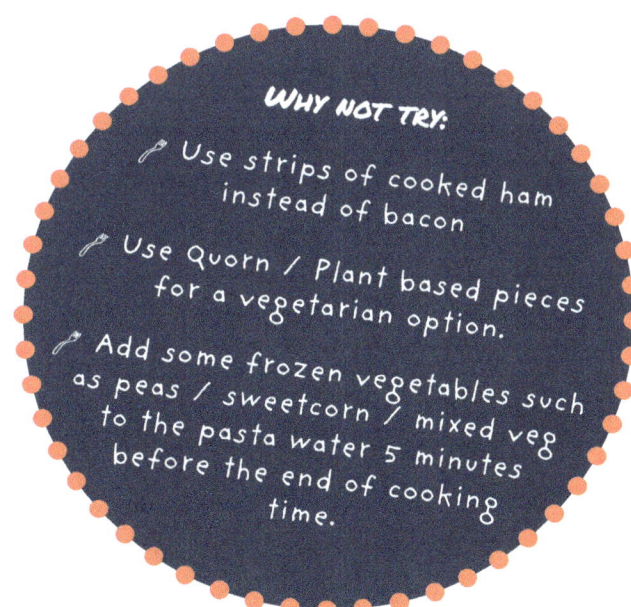

Why not try:
- Use strips of cooked ham instead of bacon
- Use Quorn / Plant based pieces for a vegetarian option.
- Add some frozen vegetables such as peas / sweetcorn / mixed veg to the pasta water 5 minutes before the end of cooking time.

Salmon Tagliatelle with Brocolli

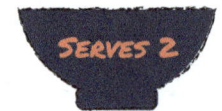

Ingredients:

Broccoli • 50g (2 large florets)
Tagliatelle (fresh or dried) • 4 sections
Salmon • 1 fillet (skin removed)
Chicken stock cubes/stock pots/Oxo • 1 dissolved in 100mls (½ mug) boiling water
Butter • 12.5g (2 teaspoons)
Spring Onion • 1 (finely sliced)
Crème Fraiche • 50mls (2 tablespoons)
Salt and Pepper

Method:

1. Put a pan of salted water on to boil.

2. Place the tagliatelle into the water and stir with a fork to separate the pasta then cook until just tender (al dente). 8-10 minutes if using dried pasta or 3 - 4 minutes if using fresh.

3. Place the salmon in a small pan, add the stock, cover and bring to the boil then simmer for 5 - 8 minutes until the salmon is just cooked and flakes easily.

4. Wash and prepare the broccoli by trimming the base of each spear and chopping into 3cm pieces.

5. Wash, trim, and slice the spring onions.

6. Transfer the salmon on to a plate and break into large flakes with a fork. Increase the heat and simmer the cooking liquid until it has reduced to about 50mls (3 tablespoons)

7. Add the butter to the reduced cooking liquid then add the spring onions and broccoli.

8. Cook for 2 - 3 minutes with the lid on then add the crème fraiche and simmer for a further 3 — 4 minutes or until the broccoli is tender.

9. Add the salmon to the pan to heat through.

10. Drain the tagliatelle in a sieve/colander and mix through the salmon mixture then serve.

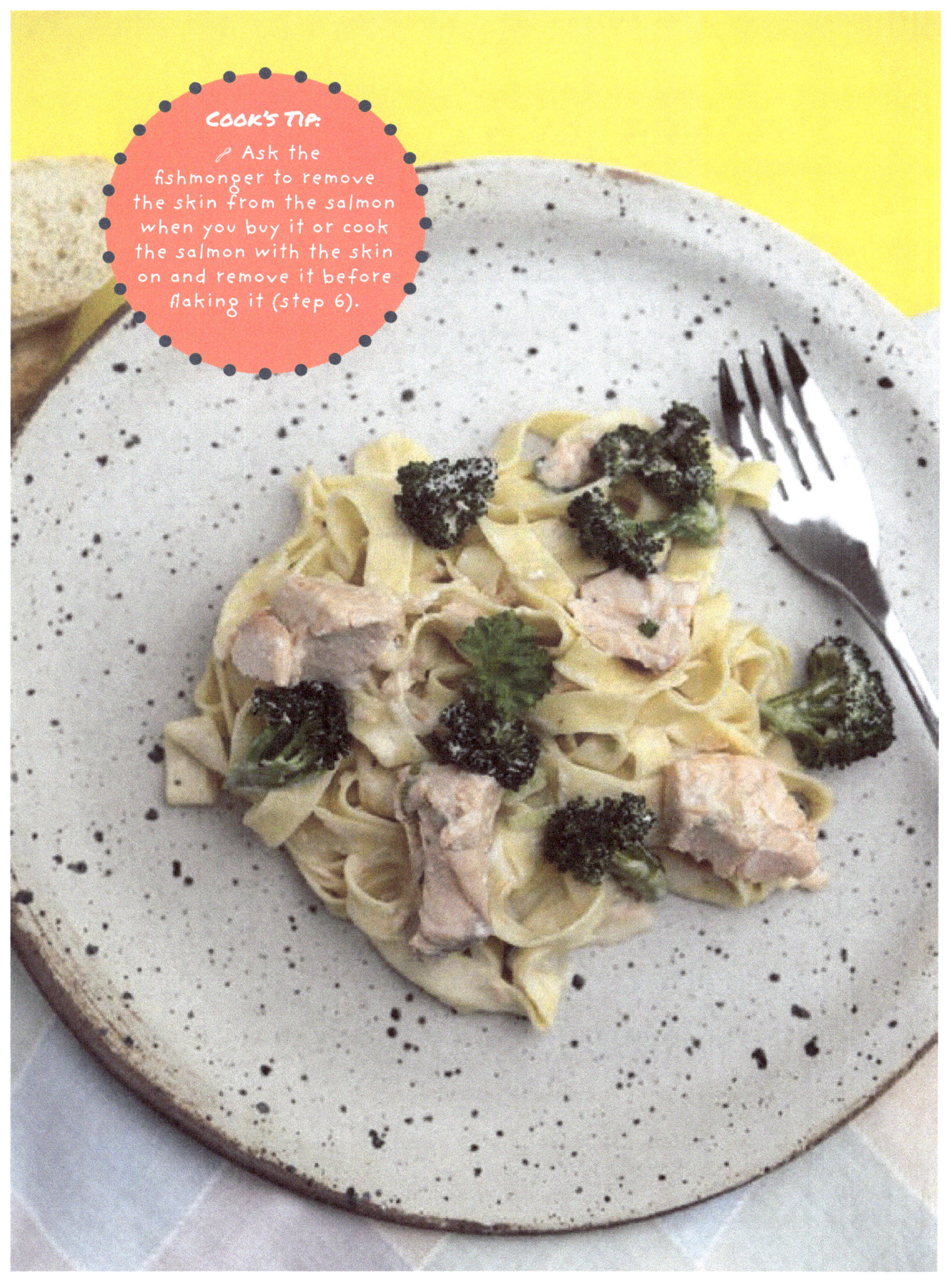

COOK'S TIP: Ask the fishmonger to remove the skin from the salmon when you buy it or cook the salmon with the skin on and remove it before flaking it (step 6).

Spicy Chicken Pasta

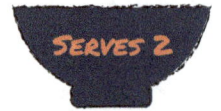

Ingredients:

Chicken Fillet (uncooked) • 2 (diced) (ask a butcher to do this for you) or 300g pack of pre-diced chicken or ½ pack (320g) of frozen diced uncooked chicken
Vegetable Oil • 5mls (1 teaspoon)
Onion • 1 small fresh or 50g (2 tablespoons) frozen/fresh ready prepared diced onion
Chicken stock cubes/stock pots • 1 dissolved in 150mls (1 mug) boiling water
Sultanas • 50g (2 tablespoons)
Frozen Peas • 50g (2 tablespoons)
Red / Green Pepper • ¼ fresh (1 tablespoon) or 1 tablespoon ready prepared or frozen mixed peppers
Curry Powder • 10 mls (2 teaspoons)
Ginger (ground) • 2.5mls (½ teaspoon)
Chilli Powder • Pinch
Chutney • 15ml (1 tablespoon)
Cornflour or Flour • 10mls (2 teaspoons)
Crème Fraiche • 30ml (2 tablespoons)
Pasta Twists/Shells/Penne • 100g (1 cup)

Method:

1. Prepare the ingredients as follows if using fresh:
   - Onion – Peel and chop
   - Garlic – Peel and crush
   - Pepper – Wash and deseed the pepper – Cut into dice
2. Dissolve the stock pot/cube in 150ml (1 mug) boiling water.
3. Heat the oil in a pan. Add the chicken and stir until it is brown all over.
4. Add the flour, curry powder, ground ginger and chilli powder and stir to coat the chicken.
5. Add the chopped onion and cook gently for a further 2 minutes.
6. Add the stock, bring to the boil and simmer gently with the lid on for 15 minutes.
7. Add the peas and red pepper and cook for a further 5 minutes.
8. Bring a pot of lightly salted water to the boil.
9. Add pasta to the boiling water and cook for 8 to 10 minutes or until al dente.
10. Add the crème fraiche and chutney to the chicken mixture Stir in well and reheat for about 1 minute.
11. Drain the pasta and rinse with boiling water.

Minestrone Pasta Pot

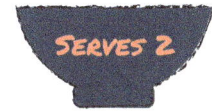

Ingredients:

Onion • ½ small fresh or 25g (1 tablespoon) frozen/fresh ready prepared diced onion
Pasta (tricolour) • 100g (1 mug)
Mixed Vegetables (frozen) • 50g (2 tablespoons)
Chopped Tomatoes (tinned) • 1 small tin (200ml) or ½ large tin
Vegetable stock cubes/stock pots • 1 dissolved in 100mls (1 cup) boiling water
Tomato Puree • 15mls (1 level tablespoon)
Baked Beans (tinned) • 1 tablespoon
Vegetable Oil • 15mls (1 tablespoon)

Serving suggestion:

Serve with some crusty, garlic or flat bread. Sprinkle the top with some grated parmesan.

Method:

1. Peel and dice onion if using fresh, and place in a frying pan with the oil.
2. Place frozen mixed vegetables on a plate.
3. Dissolve stock cube in 100mls of boiling water and then add the tinned tomatoes and tomato puree to the jug.
4. Measure pasta into a small bowl and place baked beans into a cup.
5. Sauté (gently fry) the onion for to 2-3 minutes without browning then add the pasta and contents of the jug to the pan.
6. Simmer the mixture with the pan lid on over a medium heat for 5 minutes.
7. Add the mixed vegetables to the pan and continue to simmer until pasta is almost cooked.
8. Add the baked beans to the pan and stir to heat through.
9. Turn into a serving dish.

Why not try: Add some strips of cooked ham along with the baked beans. (use Quorn/Plant based pieces for a vegetarian option).

Beef and Macaroni Bake

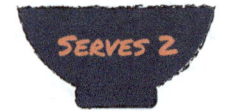

Ingredients:

Minced Beef • 250g fresh or frozen
Onion • 1 small fresh or 50g (2 tablespoons) frozen/fresh ready prepared diced onion
Garlic • 1 clove (crushed) or 2.5mls (½ teaspoon) frozen pre-chopped/lazy garlic/garlic puree/garlic powder
Chopped Tomatoes (tinned) • 1 large tin (400ml)
Beef stock cubes/stock pots/Oxo • 1 dissolved in 50mls (½ a cup) boiling water
Mushrooms • 4 large or 50g (2 tablespoons) ready prepared or frozen
Mixed Herbs (dried) • 2.5mls (½ teaspoon)
Worcestershire Sauce • 5ml (1 teaspoon)
Bay Leaf • 1
Pasta Twists/Shells/Penne • 100g (1 cup)
Salt and Pepper
Cheese (grated) • 50g (2 tablespoon) (cheddar, mozzarella or a mixture of both

Method:

1. Put oven on to Gas Mark 6 / 190°C.
2. Prepare the ingredients as follows if using fresh:
   - Onion — Peel and chop
   - Garlic — Peel and crush
   - Mushrooms — Wash and slice
3. Place mince, diced onion and garlic into a pan and brown on a high heat stirring all the time to break down the granules of mince.
4. Stir in the stock cube, chopped tomatoes, mushrooms, herbs, Worcestershire sauce and bay leaf.
5. Bring to simmering point, cover with a lid and simmer gently for approximately 20 minutes (add a little water if the mixture becomes too dry).
6. Bring a pot of lightly salted water to the boil.
7. Add pasta to the boiling water and cook for 8 to 10 minutes or until al dente.
8. Drain pasta when ready.
9. Remove the bay leaf from the meat and place the meat into a casserole dish.
10. Place the pasta over the top of the meat. Sprinkle with the grated cheese
11. Bake for 10 minutes until the cheese has browned.

Arrabiata Pasta Sauce

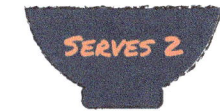
Serves 2

Ingredients:

Vegetable Oil · 15mls (1 tablespoon)
Garlic · 1 clove (crushed) or 2.5mls (½ teaspoon) frozen pre-chopped/lazy garlic/garlic puree/garlic powder
Onion · 1 small fresh or 50g (2 tablespoons) frozen/fresh ready prepared diced onion
Chopped Tomatoes (tinned) · 1 small tin (200ml) or ½ large tin
Tomato Ketchup · 5mls (1 teaspoon)
Tomato Puree · 15mls (1 level tablespoon)
Vegetable stock cubes/stock pots · 1 dissolved in 100mls (1 cup) boiling water
Sugar · 2.5mls (½ teaspoon)
Chilli flakes · Pinch
Thyme (dried) · 1.25ml (¼ teaspoon)
Basil · 2.5mls (½ teaspoon) or 1.25mls dried (¼ teaspoon)
Pasta Twists/Shells/Penne · 100g (1 mug)
Salt and Pepper

For serving:
Parmesan Cheese · 5mls (1 teaspoon)

Method:

1. Bring a pot of lightly salted water to the boil.
2. Add pasta to the boiling water and cook for 8 to 10 minutes or until al dente.
3. Prepare the onion and garlic if using fresh.
4. Make up stock in jug and add chopped tomatoes, tomato puree, ketchup and sugar.
5. Add the sugar, chilli flakes, thyme and basil to the jug.
6. Heat the oil in a frying pan and sauté (gently fry) the onion and garlic until soft.
7. Add contents of the jug and add a little salt and pepper.
8. Bring to the boil then reduce heat and simmer for 20minutes until mixture thickens.
9. Drain the pasta.
10. Remove sauce from heat and check seasoning. Then, stir the cooked pasta into the tomato sauce.
11. Transfer to serving dish and sprinkle parmesan cheese over the top.

Why Not Try:

- Saute a couple of tablespoons of chopped mixed peppers with the onion and garlic.
- Add some cooked chicken or prawns to the sauce or frozen mixed vegetables to the sauce and heat through until piping hot before adding the pasta.

All-in-One Mince and Pasta

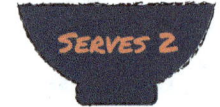

Ingredients:

Minced Beef • 250g fresh OR frozen
Onion • 1 small fresh OR 50g (2 tablespoons) frozen/fresh ready prepared diced onion
Red / Green Pepper • ½ fresh or 50g (2 tablespoons) ready prepared or frozen mixed peppers
Tomato Puree • 15mls (1 level tablespoon)
Chopped Tomatoes (tinned) • 1 small tin (200ml) or ½ large tin
Mushrooms • 2-3 fresh OR 2 tablespoons tinned or frozen sliced mushrooms (optional)
Mixed Herbs (dried) • 2.5mls (½ teaspoon)
Garlic • 1 clove (crushed) OR 2.5mls (½ teaspoon) frozen pre-chopped/lazy garlic/garlic puree/garlic powder
Beef stock cubes/stock pots/Oxo • 1 dissolved in 150mls (½ a mug) boiling water
Tomato Ketchup • 5mls (1 teaspoon)
Sugar • Pinch
Pasta Twists OR Shells • 100g (1 mug)

Method:

1. Peel and chop onion if using fresh.
2. Wash and de-seed pepper if using fresh and dice.
3. Dissolve the stock cube in the boiling water in a jug.
4. Add all the rest of the ingredients to the jug including the pasta.
5. Place mince, diced onion, and pepper into a pan.
6. Brown the mince and vegetables in the pan, stirring all the time to break down the granules of mince.
7. Stir in all the other ingredients (ie. contents of the jug).
8. Bring to simmering point, cover with a lid and simmer gently for approximately 20 minutes until the pasta is soft.
9. Stir half way through and add a little more boiling water if it's beginning to dry out and the pasta isn't soft.
10. Check seasoning. When it's ready the pasta should be soft and the liquid should be absorbed to give a sauce.

Curried Beef and Tomato Pasta

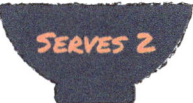

Ingredients:

Minced Beef • 250g fresh or frozen
Onion • 1 small fresh OR 50g (2 tablespoons) frozen/fresh ready prepared diced onion
Red / Green Pepper • ½ fresh or 50g (2 tablespoons) ready prepared or frozen mixed peppers
Garlic • 1 clove (crushed) OR 2.5mls (½ teaspoon) frozen pre-chopped/lazy garlic/garlic puree/garlic powder
Curry Powder • 5mls (1 teaspoon)
Chopped Tomatoes (tinned) • 1 small tin (200ml) OR ½ large tin
Tomato Soup • 1 tin (400g)
Basil (dried) • 1.25mls (¼ teaspoon)
Pasta Twists/Shells/Penne • 100g (1 cup)
Salt and Pepper

Method:

1. Prepare the ingredients as follows if using fresh:
   - Onion — Peel and chop
   - Pepper — Wash, deseed and slice
   - Garlic — Peel and crush

2. Place mince into a pan and brown on a high heat stirring all the time to break down the granules of mince.

3. Add the garlic, onion, red/green pepper, dried basil and curry powder to the pan and cook for 1 minute.

4. Add the tinned tomatoes, tomato soup and pasta and bring to the boil.

5. Simmer with a lid on for 15 minutes until the pasta is tender (add a little water if the mixture becomes too dry).

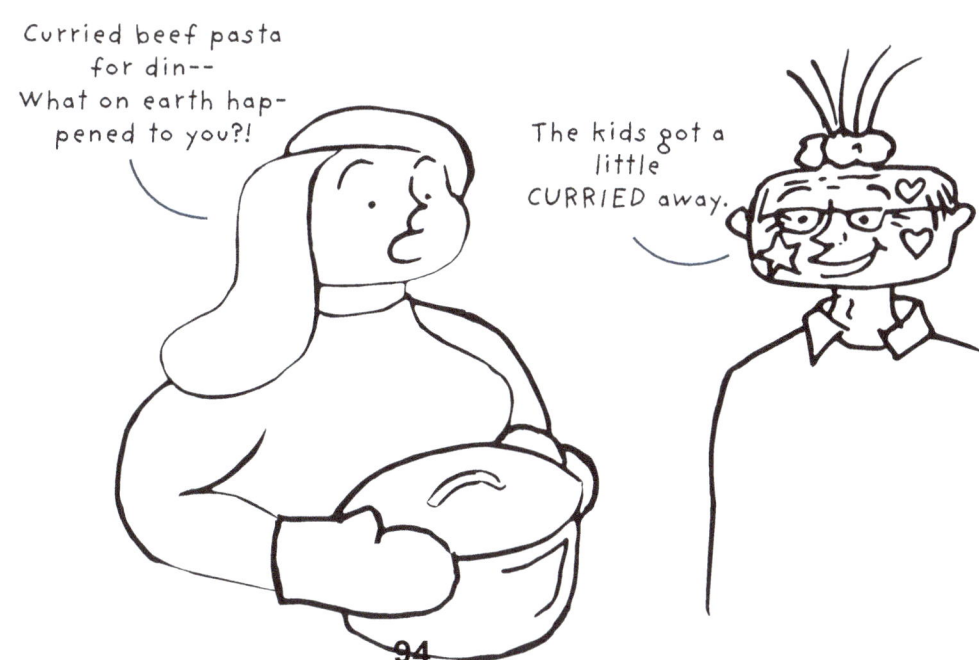

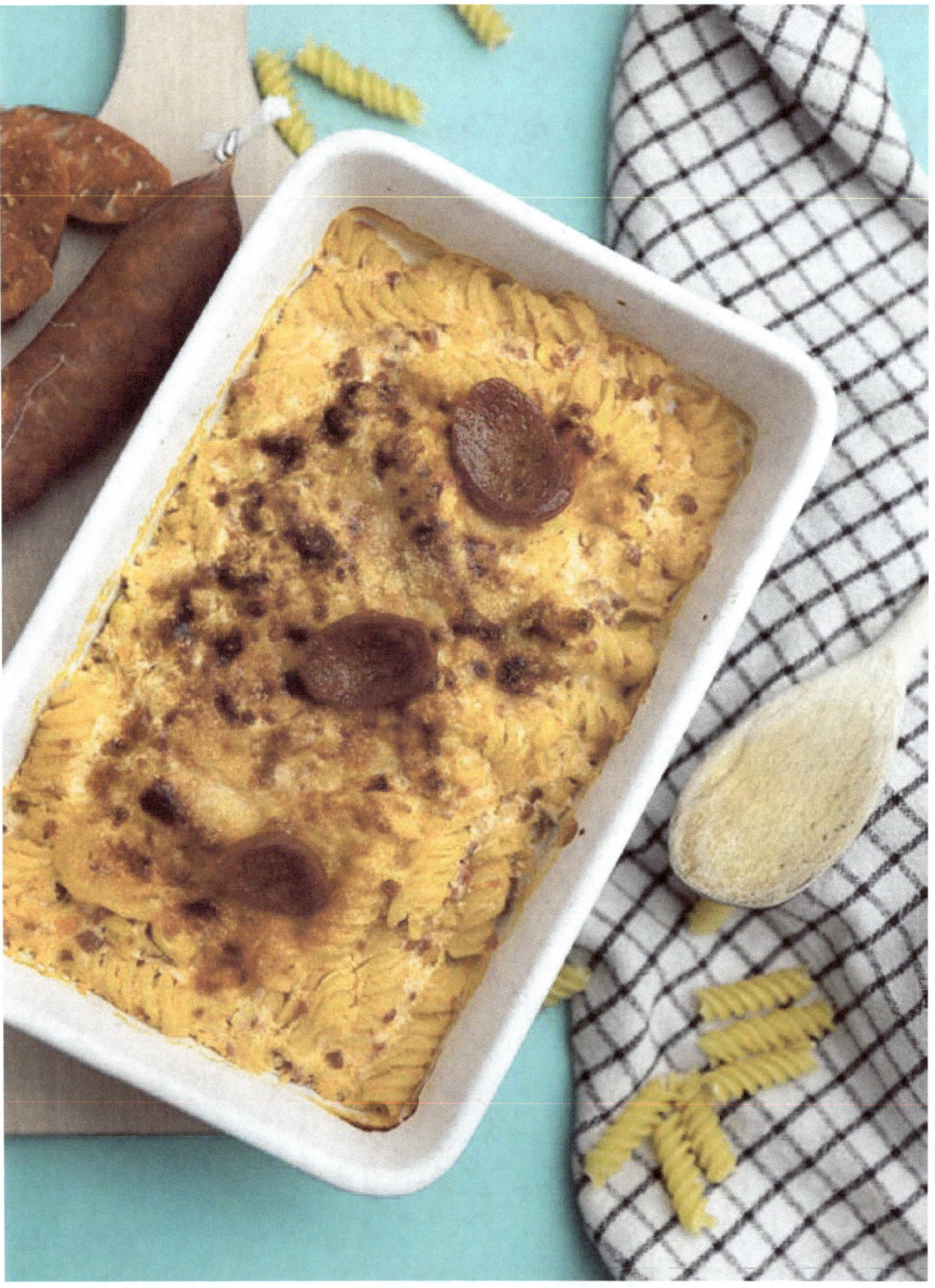

Chorizo and Sweetcorn Pasta Bake

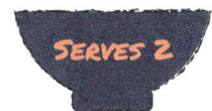

Ingredients:

Pasta Twists/Shells/Penne - 100g (1 cup)
Vegetable Oil - 5ml (1 teaspoon)
Chorizo (cooked and diced) - ½ pack (65g) or ¼ of a fresh cooked chorizo sausage / ¼ of a pack of frozen diced chorizo
Frozen Sweetcorn - 50g (2 tablespoons)
Garlic - 1 clove (crushed) or 2.5mls (½ teaspoon) frozen pre-chopped/lazy garlic/garlic puree/garlic powder
Ricotta Cheese - 250g tub
Milk - 100ml (1 cup)
Parmesan (grated) — 25g (1 tablespoon)
Salt and Pepper

Method:

1. Put on the oven Gas mark 6, 200°C/190°C fan oven
2. Prepare the ingredients
   - Peel and crush the garlic
   - Cut the chorizo into slices and then into small dice
3. Half fill saucepan with cold water, add ½ teaspoon of salt. Put on to boil.
4. When the water boils add the penne, boil for about 15 minutes until the just tender Drain.
5. Gently heat a pan with the oil in it and gently fry the garlic and chorizo for about 2 minutes.
6. Mix the ricotta cheese and the milk.
7. Add the penne, sweetcorn and ricotta cheese to the pan and mix. Taste for seasoning.
8. Place in a casserole dish, sprinkle with the grated parmesan cheese and bake for 15-20 minutes until golden brown

Cook's Tip:

- If you don't have any penne pasta, any other type can be used
- The chorizo can be dry fried without any additional oil

Pasta Carbonara

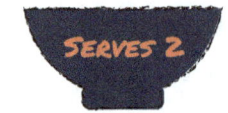

Ingredients:

Spaghetti / Pasta Shapes • 100g
Lardons • 1 small pack (unsmoked) OR 1-2 rasher unsmoked back bacon (chopped)
Vegetable Oil • 5ml (1 teaspoon)
Soft Cream Cheese • 100g (½ a tub)
Milk • 50ml (2 tablespoons)
Parmesan (grated) • 50g (2 tablespoons)
Garlic • 1 clove (crushed) OR 2.5mls (½ teaspoon) frozen pre-chopped/lazy garlic/garlic puree/garlic powder
Salt and Pepper

Serving Suggestion:

Serve with some hot crusty or garlic bread

Method:

1. Half fill a pan with water, add ½ teaspoon salt and bring to the boil

2. Add pasta to the boiling water and simmer for approx 15 minutes. Drain when ready.

3. Prepare ingredients:
   - Using the scissors, cut the bacon into small pieces.
   - Peel and crush the garlic

4. Heat the olive oil gently, add the bacon and cook for about 2 – 3 minutes until ready.

5. Add the garlic, milk, cream cheese and ½ the parmesan cheese into the pan. Simmer gently over a low heat until the cheese has melted. Simmer for 1 minute.

6. Add the drained pasta to the sauce. Mix gently.

7. Place into a dish and sprinkle the remaining parmesan cheese on top. Serve.

Why Not Try:

- Add some sliced mushrooms and cook with the lardons/bacon
- Use Quorn / Plant based rashers for a vegetarian option.

Desserts

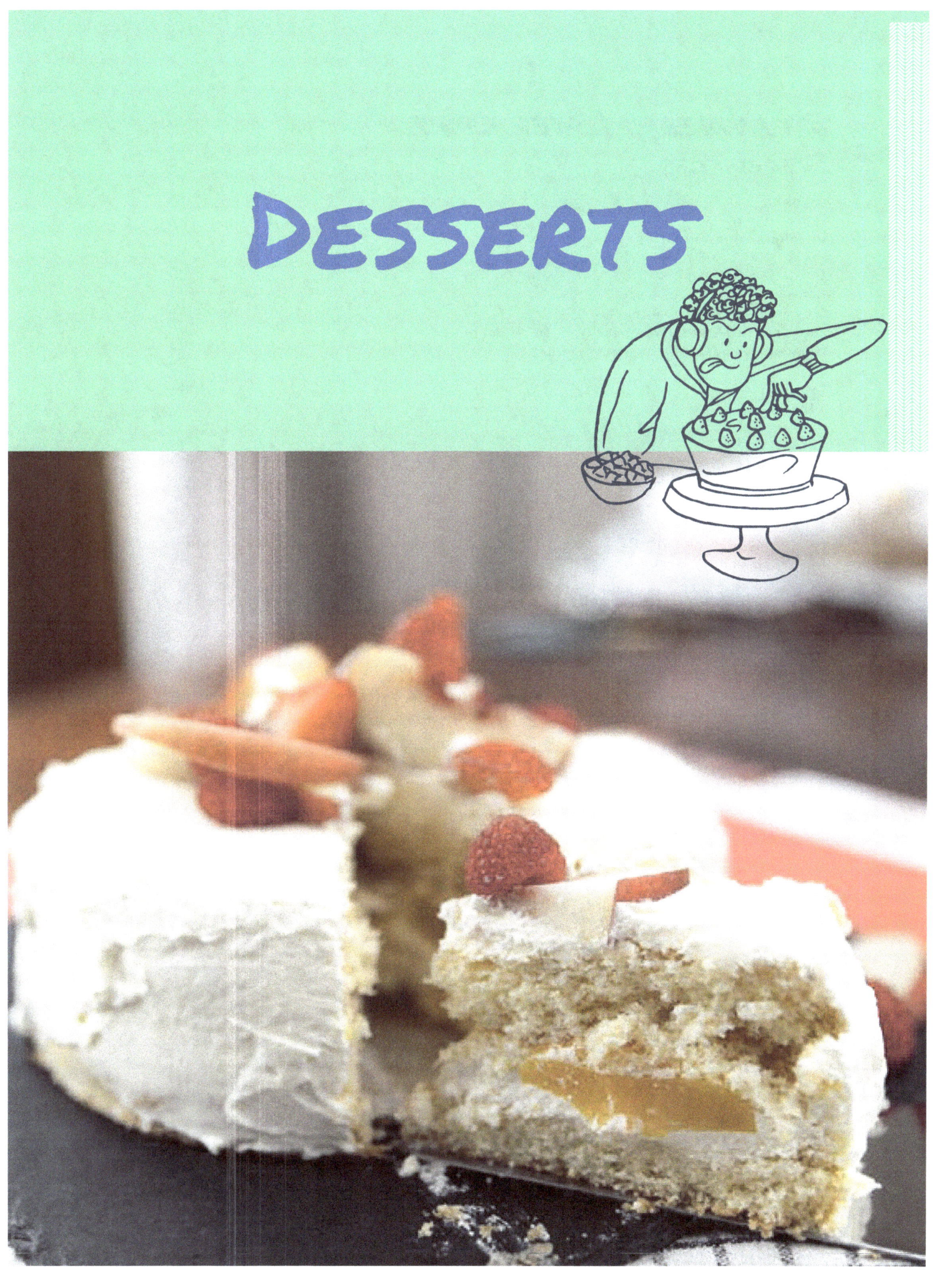

Strawberry Layer Cake

Ingredients:

Sponge:
Caster sugar · 50g
Self-Raising Flour · 50g
Eggs · 2 at room temperature

Filling:
Cream (double) · 150ml carton
Yoghurt (thick set strawberry) · 1 small carton
Strawberries (fresh) · a small punnet

Topping:
Icing sugar

Method:

1. Set oven to Gas Mark 5, 190°C.
2. Grease and line a Swiss roll tin with greaseproof paper (see Kitchen Journal). Sieve flour on to a plate.
3. Whisk eggs and sugar in a bowl until light and fluffy (the mixture should resemble whipped cream)
4. Carefully fold in the sieved flour.
5. Turn the mixture into the greased tin and bake for 10-15 minutes until golden brown and springs back when touched.
6. Whisk the cream until mixture holds peaks (do not over whip as cream will turn to butter). Then fold the yoghurt into the cream.
7. Remove the sponge from the oven, turn on to a cooling tray and remove the greaseproof paper. Set to one side to cool.
8. Wash and dry the strawberries, remove the stalks and slice.
9. Carefully trim the two short edges off the sponge and then cut it into three equal pieces.
10. Place one piece of the sponge on to a plate then spread half of strawberry yoghurt mixture over the surface and place half of the sliced strawberries over the top of yoghurt mixture.
11. Place a second piece of the cake on top of this and repeat with the rest of the yoghurt mixture and strawberries.
12. Place the third layer of the cake over the top of this and sieve a thin layer of icing sugar over the top.

Chocolate Layer Cake

Ingredients:

Sponge:
Caster sugar · 50g
Self-Raising Flour · 50g
Eggs · 2 at room temperature
Drinking Chocolate · 1 level tablespoon

Filling
Cream (double) · 150ml carton

Topping
Icing sugar

Method:

1. Set oven to Gas Mark 5, 190°C.
2. Grease and line a Swiss roll tin with greaseproof paper (see Kitchen Journal).
3. Sieve the flour and drinking chocolate on to a plate.
4. Whisk eggs and sugar in a bowl until light and fluffy (the mixture should resemble whipped cream)
5. Carefully fold in the sieved flour and chocolate powder.
6. Turn the mixture into the greased tin and bake for 10-15 minutes until golden brown and springs back when touched.
7. Whisk the cream until mixture holds peaks (do not over whip as cream will turn to butter).
8. Remove the sponge from the oven, turn on to a cooling tray and remove the greaseproof paper. Set to one side to cool.
9. Carefully trim the two short edges off the sponge and then cut it into three equal pieces.
10. Place one piece of the sponge on to a plate then spread half of the cream over the surface.
11. Place a second piece of the cake on top of this and repeat with the rest of the cream.
12. Place the last layer of the cake over the top of this and sieve a thin layer of icing sugar over the top.

Vanilla Panna Cotta

Ingredients:

Cream (double) · 350mls
Milk · 150mls
Caster Sugar · 65g (2 good tablespoons)
Vanilla Paste · 15mls
Gelatine · 2 sheets

Method:

1. Place the gelatine in a bowl of cold water to soften.
2. Place vanilla paste in a pan with the milk and cream. Then add the sugar to the pan and bring to a simmer and the sugar is dissolved.
3. Whilst the cream mixture is still hot, remove the softened gelatine from the water, squeeze out the water then whisk into the cream mixture to dissolve.
4. Place the mixture into a bowl and place this bowl over a bowl of ice to allow the mixture to cool quicker.
5. Stir the mixture every so often to make sure the vanilla is well mixed through it.
6. Once the mixture has started to set transfer it to a serving dish and refrigerate until fully set.

Coriander, Lemongrass, and Pineapple Compote

Ingredients:

Pineapple (fresh) · ½ (diced)
Lemongrass · 1 (bashed)
Coriander leaf (fresh) · 15mls (chopped)
Stock Syrup · 200mls (see method below)

Serving Suggestions:

Spoon the pineapple compote over the top of the set Panna Cotta.

Method:

1. Make the stock syrup by placing 200mls water and 200g sugar in a pan and bringing to the boil. Once the sugar has dissolved add the bashed lemongrass and simmer for 2-3 minutes. Remove from the heat and allow to infuse.
2.
3.
4. Peel and dice the pineapple and chop the coriander.
5. Place the pineapple into a hot frying pan and sauté (lightly fry) for a few minutes. Add a couple of turns of black pepper to the pan then add the infused stock syrup 2-3 tablespoons at a time until you get a syrup compote.
6.
7. Allow syrup to cool and add a large pinch of the freshly chopped coriander.

Place in fridge to cool.

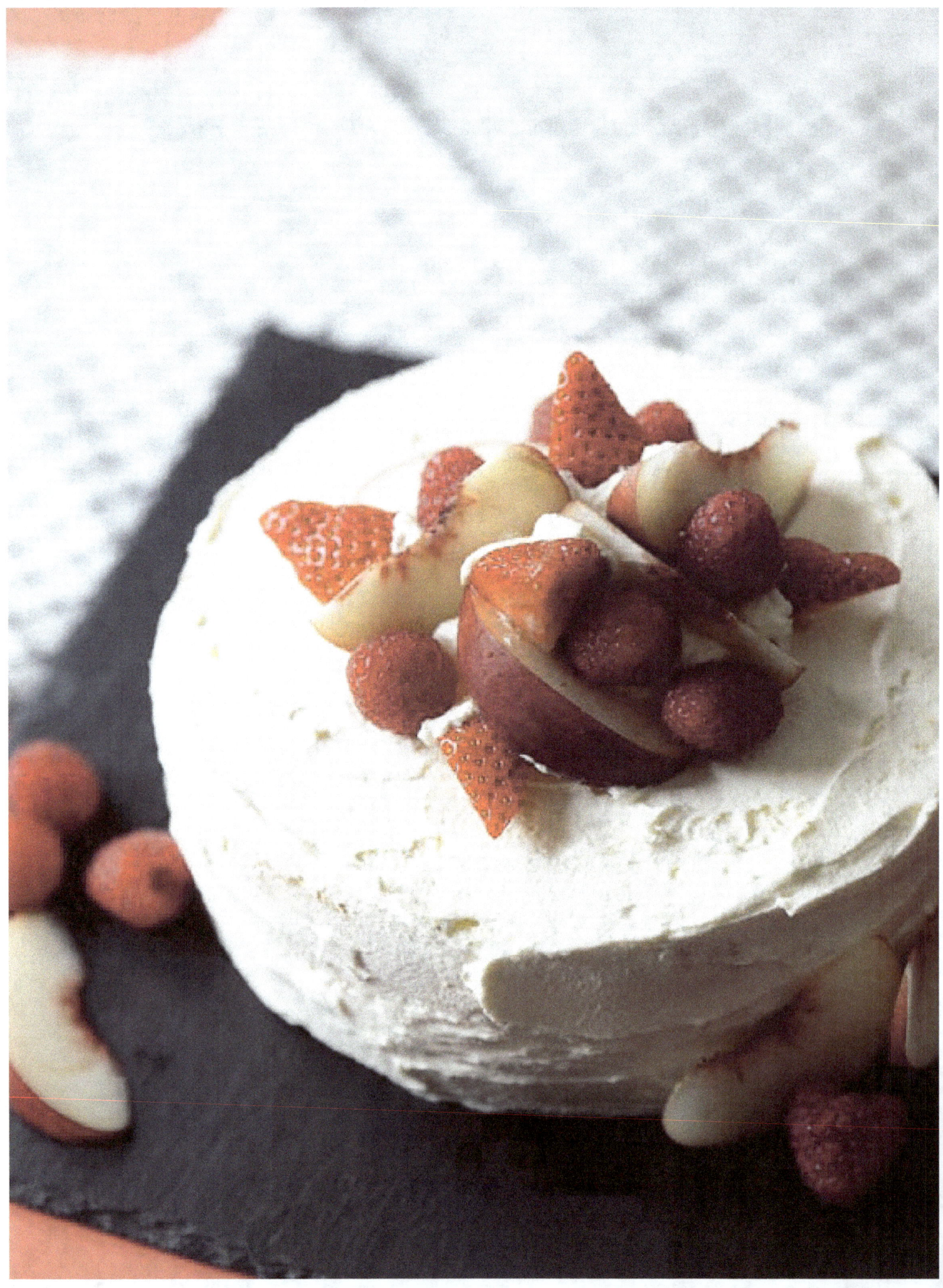

Mandarin or Peach Gateau

Ingredients:

Sponge:
Caster sugar · 75g
Self-Raising Flour · 75g
Eggs · 3 at room temperature

Filling:
Cream (double) · 300ml carton
Yoghurt (thick set mandarin/peach) · 1 small carton
Mandarin Oranges OR Peaches in juice · 1 tin (drained)

Decoration:
Small packet chocolate buttons
Piped cream (optional)
Other ½ tin mandarin oranges OR peaches (drained)

Why Not Try: Make the sponge chocolate by replacing 1 dessertspoonful of the sieved flour with the same amount of cocoa powder.

Method:

1. Set oven to Gas Mark 5, 190°C.
2. Grease and line two sandwich tins with greaseproof paper (see Kitchen Journal)
3. Sieve flour on to a plate.
4. Whisk eggs and sugar in a clean bowl until light and fluffy (should leave a trail on the surface).
5. Carefully fold in the sieved flour.
6. Divide mixture evenly between the two cake tins and bake for 15-20 minutes until sponges spring back when touched.
7. Allow sponges to cool slightly then run a sharp knife around the inside edge of the tin and turn the sponges out.
8. Remove greaseproof paper and cool on a wire tray.
9. Whisk cream until mixture holds peaks.
10. Place ½ of the cream into a small bowl and stir in the yoghurt.
11. Assemble the two sponges with the yoghurt cream and the ½ tin of drained fruit.
12. Decorate with the rest of the fruit, some piped cream and chocolate buttons.

Easy Fruity Yoghurt Dessert

Ingredients:

Cream (double) · 300ml carton
Yoghurt (thick set blueberry) · 3 small cartons (see other suggestions below)
Yoghurt (thick set Natural) · 1 small carton
Blueberries (fresh) · 150g tub

Method:

1. Whisk the cream to soft peak consistency.
2. Add the 3 fruit and 1 natural yoghurts to the cream.
3. Carefully whisk the yoghurts into the cream (the mixture should still be thick and creamy).
4. Stir in the blueberries.
5. Transfer to a serving dish.
6. Sprinkle soft brown sugar lightly over the surface and refrigerate.

> **Why Not Try:**
> - Use other flavoured yoghurts and fruit such as Strawberry or Raspberry.
> - Use Fudge/Toffee yoghurt and instead of using fruit crush a couple of Crunchies and stir them through the yoghurt mixture.

Eton Mess

Ingredients:

Cream (double) · 300ml carton
Strawberries (fresh) · a small punnet
Meringue nests · 4 or 6 meringue shells

Method:

1. Cut the strawberries in half or into thick slices if they're big.
2. Whisk the cream until it forms soft peaks.
3. Fold the strawberries into the cream.
4. Crush the meringues and fold them into the strawberry and cream mixture.
5. Spoon the Eton mess into individual dishes.

Chilled Lemon Flan

Ingredients:

Base:
Digestive Biscuits · 100g
Margarine · 50g

Filling:
Lemon · 1 small
Condensed milk · ½ tin of (200g)
Cream (double) · 150ml carton

Decoration:
Additional whipped cream for piping (optional)
Mini marshmallows/white chocolate buttons

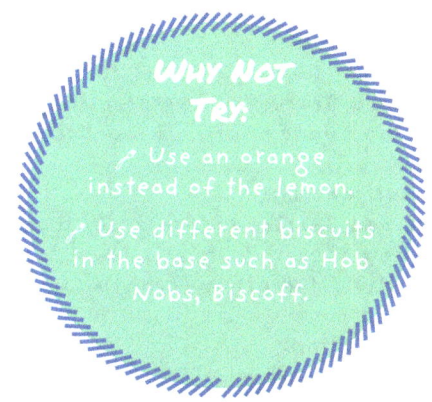

Why Not Try:
- Use an orange instead of the lemon.
- Use different biscuits in the base such as Hob Nobs, Biscoff.

Method:

1. Crush biscuits for base in a food processor or place in a polythene bag and crush with a rolling pin.

2. Melt margarine in pan, remove from heat and stir in biscuits.

3. Place biscuit mixture into a flan dish/sandwich tin and flatten down with the back of a metal spoon.

4. Place biscuit base in the fridge to chill.

5. Wash lemon, grate zest and squeeze juice of lemon.

6. Whip cream in a bowl to a piping consistency (do not over whip).

7. Pour the condensed milk, lemon juice and lemon zest into a large bowl and beat until smooth.

8. Carefully fold the cream into the lemon mixture and spoon over the biscuit base.

   Optional: Pipe a border of cream around edge of the flan and decorate with the mini marshmallows / chocolate buttons.

Mixed Berry Shortcake

Ingredients:

Shortcake:
Plain Flour · 100g
Butter or Margarine (softened) · 100g
Cornflour · 50g
Icing Sugar · 50g

Fruit Cream:
Cream (double) · 150ml carton
Mixed Berry Fruits (selection) · 100g
Icing Sugar · 15mls (1 level tablespoon)

Fruit Coulis:
Mixed Berries (fresh) · 100g or 100g frozen (defrosted)
Icing Sugar · 30mls (2 level tablespoons)
Water (if fruit is fresh) · 20mls

Decoration:
Whipped cream
Icing sugar for dusting

Method:

1. Set oven to Gas Mark 4, 180°C.
2. Place all the ingredients for the shortcake into a food processor and mix until dough comes together.
3. Turn mixture out on to a lightly floured table top, knead lightly until smooth and roll out to approximately 3mm.
4. Cut biscuits out using cutter and place on baking tray.
5. Bake until golden brown.
6. Allow to cool slightly before removing from baking tray as biscuits will still be soft.

Fruit Cream:

7. Pureé the mixed berries then pass through a sieve to remove any seeds.
8. Whisk the double cream until stiff.
9. Fold the mixed berries and icing sugar into the whipped cream until evenly mixed.
10. Cover and refrigerate until required.

Fruit Coulis:

11. Pureé the fruit for the coulis then pass through a sieve to remove the seeds.
12. Add the icing sugar and water (if required) and stir until all the sugar has dissolved and the coulis has a smooth consistency.
13. Cover and chill until required.

Assembling:

14. Sandwich two of the shortcake biscuits together with the fruit cream and place on serving dish.
15. Dust lightly with icing sugar.
16. Carefully pour a little of the coulis around each shortcake.
17. Decorate if desired with piped rosettes of cream, raspberries/strawberries and/or any other decorations.

Sticky Toffee Pudding

Ingredients:

Sticky Toffee Pudding:
Caster sugar · 110g
Self-Raising Flour · 100g (sieved)
Margarine · 30g
Eggs · 1 at room temperature
Date Pieces · 100g (optional)
Water · 150mls
Bicarbonate of Soda · 1.25mls (¼ teaspoon)
Vanilla Essence · 1.25mls (¼ teaspoon)

Butterscotch Sauce:
Cream (double) · 125ml
Butter · 30g
Demerara Sugar · 50g (2 tablespoons)

Decoration:
Additional whipped cream (optional)

Serving Suggestions:

Divide into equal portions and serve with a decoration of rosettes/spoonful of cream.

To reheat microwave until piping hot.

Method:

1. Set oven to Gas Mark 5, 190°C.
2. Grease an 18cm sandwich tin.
3. Boil the dates in the water for approximately 5 minutes until soft then add the bicarbonate of soda. Remove from the heat and cool slightly.
4. Cream the butter and sugar for the pudding together until light and fluffy then gradually beat in the egg.
5. Fold in the dates, flour and vanilla essence.
6. Place mixture into the greased tin and bake for 30-40 minutes until firm to touch.
7. Place cream for sauce into a pan and bring to the boil then whisk in the butter and sugar. Simmer for 3 minutes.
8. Sauce can be poured over the top of the sticky toffee pudding or reserved and served separately.

Apple & Cinammon Parcels

Ingredients:

Cooking Apple - 350g (1 large)
Soft Brown Sugar - 50g (2 tablespoons)
Plain Flour - 25g (1 tablespoon)
Cinnamon - 2.5mls (½ teaspoon)
Butter (unsalted) - 50g
Filo Pastry - 1 pack

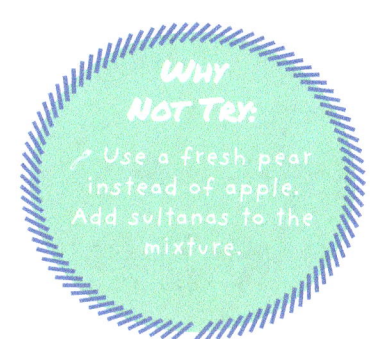

Why Not Try:
Use a fresh pear instead of apple.
Add sultanas to the mixture.

Method:

1. Set oven to Gas Mark 5, 190°C.
2. Peel and grate the apples then coat in the flour, cinnamon, and brown sugar.
3. Melt the butter in either a pan or in a bowl in the microwave.
4. Cut the filo pastry into rectangles, 6cm by 18cm and stack one on top of the other.
5. Refer to following diagrams below to help assemble the parcels.

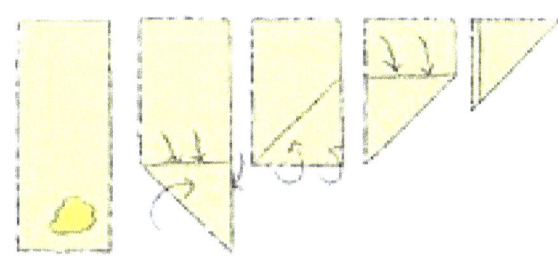

fig.1   fig.2   fig.3   fig.4   fig.5

6. Lightly butter the edges of the top triangle.
7. Place a teaspoon of the apple mixture into each parcel (see figure 1).
8. Fold the bottom left hand corner over the filling to make a triangle shape and seal the edges (see figure 2).
9. Fold the right hand point up keeping the triangle shape and press in the edges to seal again. Continue folding left then right sealing as you go until the end of the rectangle of pastry.
10. Place on a baking tray then repeat the above stages with each of the triangles.
11. Bake for 10 minutes until golden brown.
12. Dust with icing sugar and serve.

Fruit Kebab with Chocolate Dip

Ingredients:

Kebabs:
Orange · 1
Peach or Nectarine · 1
Kiwi Fruit · 1
Grapes green and/or black · a handful OR 1/2 cup
Strawberries (fresh) · a handful OR 1/2 cup

Dip:
Chocolate Spread · 1 tablespoon
Milk · 1 tablespoon

Method:

1. Prepare fruits for the kebabs by washing, peeling where required and cutting into even sized pieces.

2. Thread fruits on to cocktail sticks and place to one side

3. For the dip place the chocolate spread and milk into a microwave-safe dish and heat through to melt.

4. Pour sauce over fruit kebabs or serve it in a small jug/ramekin on the side.

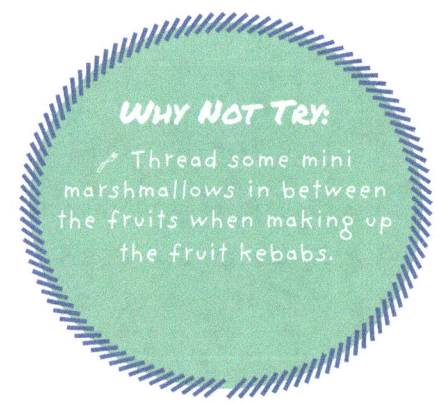

Why Not Try:
Thread some mini marshmallows in between the fruits when making up the fruit kebabs.

White Chocolate & Lime Cheesecake

Ingredients:

Ginger Nut Biscuits · 100g
Butter · 40g
Lime · 1
Cream Cheese · 100g
Caster Sugar · 20g
Cream (double) · 150ml carton
White Cooking Chocolate · 75g

Method:

1. Crush the ginger nut biscuits.
2. Melt the butter in a pan then add the biscuits and mix.
3. Turn biscuit mixture into a small round sandwich tin and press down with the back of a metal spoon. Chill.
4. Wash and grate the rind of the lime and squeeze out the juice and keep until required.
5. Beat the cream cheese with the sugar.
6. Whisk the cream until soft peak consistency.
7. Melt the chocolate and mix with the cream cheese then add the lime zest and 15mls of the juice.
8. Fold in half of the cream, reserve the rest of the cream for decorating the cheesecake.
9. Spoon the cream cheese mixture over the biscuit base and chill.
10. Before serving pipe the remaining cream on top.

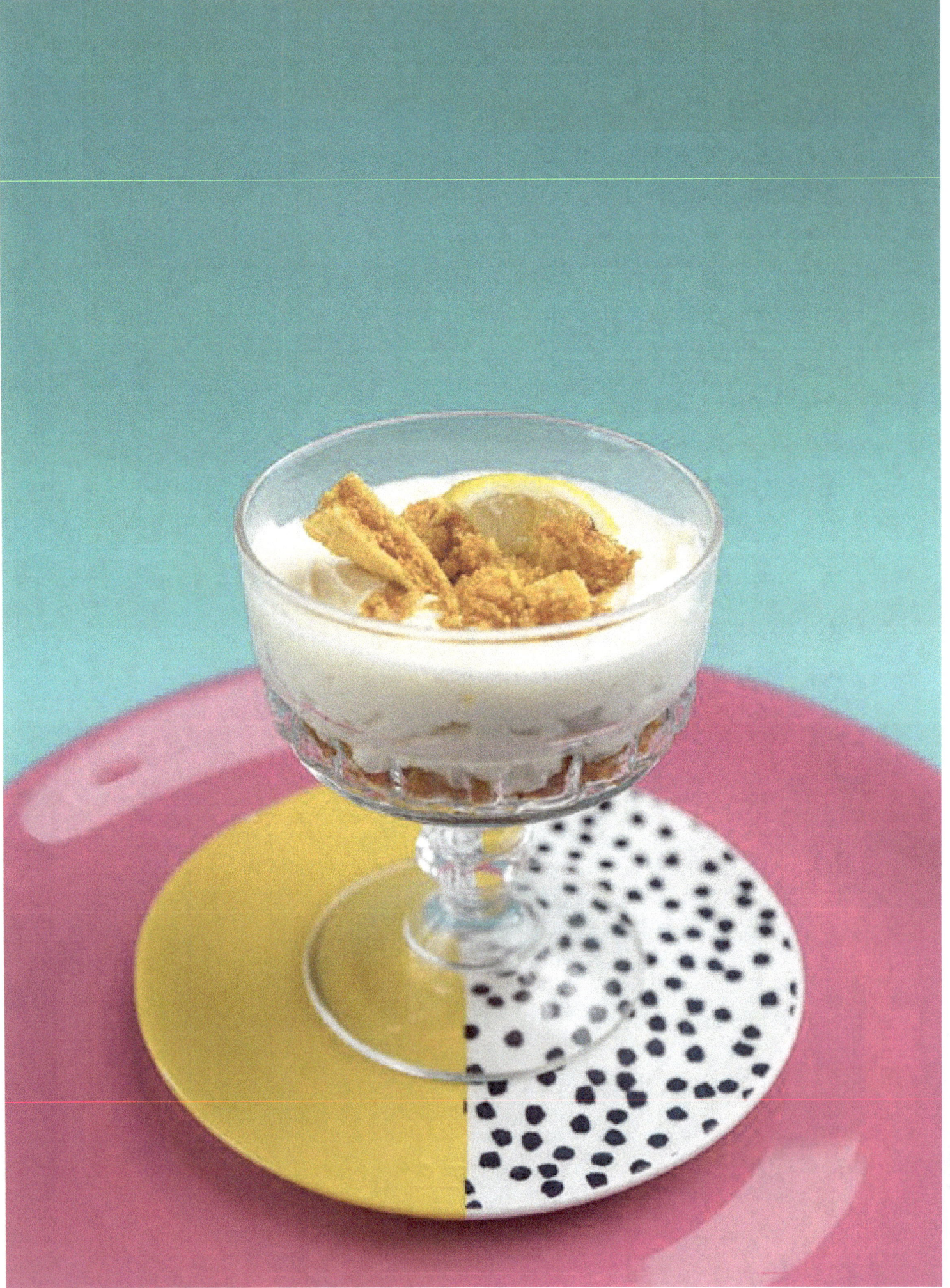

Lemon Posset with Honeycomb

Ingredients:

Cream Cheese · 200g tub
Icing Sugar · 75g (3 tablespoons)
Lemon Curd · 50g (2 tablespoons)
Cream (double) · 300ml carton
Lemon (half) · juice and rind

Honeycomb pieces · 50g (½ bag)

Serving Suggestions:

Make into individual servings and place each dish on a serving plate and decorate with some fresh redcurrants and a dusting of icing sugar.

Serve with a little Highlander shortbread or 'Biscoff' biscuit on the side.

Method:

1. Mix cream cheese, sugar, lemon curd, lemon rind and lemon juice together.
2. Whisk cream until soft peak stage.
3. Fold cream into the lemon mixture and place in the fridge to chill.
4. Place 1/3 of the honeycomb pieces into the base of a glass serving dish.
5. Carefully spoon half of the lemon posset mixture over the top.
6. Repeat this process.
7. Finish the dish with a sprinkling of honeycomb.

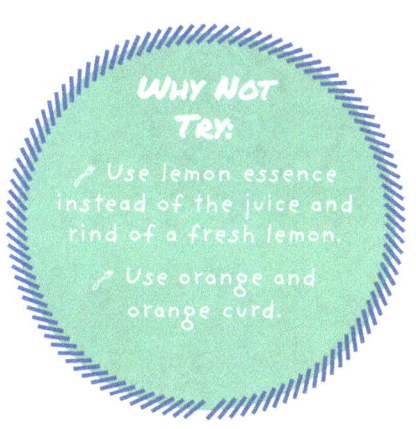

Why Not Try:
- Use lemon essence instead of the juice and rind of a fresh lemon.
- Use orange and orange curd.

Cheat's Tiramisu

Ingredients:

Custard (fresh) · 1 carton or 1 tin ready-made custard
Cream (double) · 300ml carton
Sponge Fingers · 1 packet
Coffee · 1 heaped teaspoon of dissolved in 100mls boiling water
Liqueur (Amaretto, Brandy, Dark Rum) · 2 tablespoons or water
Chocolate (Grated) / Crushed Flake · 1 tablespoon

Method:

1. Prepare the coffee and add the liqueur (if not using liqueur add the water)
2. Whip the cream to soft peak consistency and fold half into the custard.
3. Dip half the sponge fingers into the coffee mixture and place a layer in bottom of dish (don't over soak the biscuits as they will go soggy).
4. Spread half the custard mixture over the sponge fingers.
5. Dip the other half of the sponge fingers into the coffee mixture and place over the top of the custard mixture.
6. Spread the rest of the custard mixture over the sponge fingers.
7. Finish by spreading the rest of the cream over the surface and sprinkle the grated chocolate/flake over the top.
8. Chill before serving.

Cook's Tip: This dessert can be made 24 hours in advance of serving to allow the biscuits to absorb the flavours.

Fruit Crumble Tart

Ingredients:

- **Plain flour** · 100g (4 tablespoons)
- **Wholemeal Flour** · 100g (4 tablespoons)
- **Margarine** · 100g
- **Cold water** · (approx 6 teaspoons)
- **Soft Brown Sugar** · 25g (1 tablespoon)
- **Fruit Pie Filling** · 1 tin (you can choose either apple, summer fruits or black cherry)

Method:

1. Set oven to Gas Mark 6, 200°C.
2. Place flour and add margarine into a large bowl then rub it in until it resembles fine breadcrumbs (you can use a food processor for this).
3. Remove 3 tablespoons of the mixture and place it into a small bowl along with the brown sugar and stir to mix.
4. Set small bowl to one side.
5. Carefully add water a teaspoonful at a time to the mixture in the large bowl and stir with a kitchen knife until the mixture forms a stiff dough (you can also do this stage in the food processor).
6. Turn the dough out on to a lightly floured tabletop and knead until smooth.
7. Roll out the dough and use to line a sandwich tin / flan dish.
8. Pour the pie filling into the pastry case.
9. Sprinkle the crumble topping from the small bowl over the pie filling.
10. Bake for 15-20 minutes or until the top is golden brown and the pastry case is baked.

Why Not Try:

- The tin of pie filling could be changed to home-made stewed apples/rhubarb.
- Make mini tarts by cutting out pastry circles with a cutter and placing them into a patty tin, then placing a teaspoonful of pie filling into each case and finely sprinkling a teaspoonful of the crumble topping over each tart. Bake for 10-14 minutes.
- You can use a packet of shortcut pastry mix instead of making your own and skip to step 3 of the method.
- Use a sweet pastry case instead of making your own and a packet of crumble mix to top the pie filing.

Plate Apple Tart

Ingredients:

Pastry:
Plain Flour · 200g
Margarine · 100g
Cold water to mix

Filling:
Apple Pie Filling · 1 tin

Glaze:
Milk · 1 tablespoon
Caster Sugar · 2 tablespoons

Alternatives are:
- 450g packet of shortcrust pastry mix
- 500g packet of pre-made
- Ready rolled shortcrust pastry

Method:

1. Set oven to Gas Mark 6, 200°C.
2. If making your own pastry sieve the flour into large bowl and rub in margarine until mixture resembles fine breadcrumbs
3. Add enough cold water a teaspoon at a time to make a firm dough (you could use a food processor to make the pastry)
4. Turn pastry on to a lightly floured work surface and knead lightly.
5. Divide pastry into 3.
6. Roll one of the pieces into a circle for the lid.
7. Put the other two pieces of pastry together and knead lightly until smooth and roll out and use to line a sandwich tin / flan dish.
8. Pour the apple pie filling into the case then dampen the edges of the pastry with a little cold water.
9. Place the lid over the top and seal the edges.
10. Trim any excess pastry from the edges (you can use any trimmings to make decorations for the top of tart and stick them to the lid with a little cold water).
11. Brush top of the pastry with a little milk and sprinkle with the caster sugar.
12. Bake for 20-25 minutes until pastry is golden brown

Fruity Bread Pudding

Ingredients:

Bread · 100g (4 slices)
Apple Juice · 250ml
Mixed Dried Fruit · 75g (3 tablespoons)
Cinnamon or Mixed Spice · 5ml (1 teaspoon)
Banana · 1
Milk · 150ml
Eggs · 1
Brown Sugar · 25g (1 tablespoon)

Method:

1. Set oven to Gas Mark 6, 200°C.
2. Cut or tear the bread into small pieces approximately 1 cm dice.
3. Thinly slice the banana.
4. Place the dried fruit, apple juice and cinnamon/mixed spice into a pan and bring to the boil.
5. Remove the pan from the heat and allow to cool slightly
6. Place the bread and banana in the base of a greased ovenproof dish.
7. Beat the egg and milk together and add to the apple juice and fruit mixture.
8. Pour the liquid over the bread and sprinkle the brown sugar on top
9. Bake in the oven until golden brown

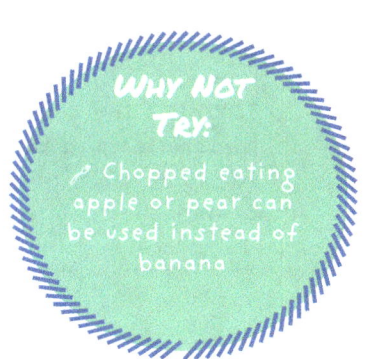

Why Not Try:
- Chopped eating apple or pear can be used instead of banana

Apple Crumble

Ingredients:

Crumble topping:
Plain/Wholemeal Flour • 3 tablespoons
Porridge Oats/Oatmeal • 1 tablespoon
Coconut/Muesli • 1 tablespoon
Soft Brown Sugar • 1 tablespoon
Margarine • 1 heaped tablespoon

Filling:
Apple Slices • 1 tin (drained)
Sultanas • 1 tablespoon
Soft Brown Sugar • 1 teaspoon
Cinnamon, Mixed Spice or Ginger • 1.25mls (¼ teaspoon) (optional)

Method:

1. Set oven to Gas mark 5, 190°C.
2. Place flour into a large bowl.
3. Add the margarine to the bowl and rub in with the fingers until the mixture resembles fine breadcrumbs (you can use a food processor for this).
4. Add the porridge oats, coconut and brown sugar for the crumble topping to the bowl and mix. Set to one side.
5. Place the apples for the filling into a small bowl and cut up into slightly smaller pieces.
6. Add the sultanas, teaspoon of brown sugar and cinnamon to the bowl and stir to mix.
7. Turn the apple mixture into an ovenproof dish.
8. Sprinkle the crumble topping over the apples and bake in the oven for 15 – 20 minutes until golden brown.

Why Not Try:

- The apples can be changed to another type of tinned fruit such as peaches, pineapple, rhubarb, raspberries.
- Any frozen fruit eg. summer fruits, raspberries, strawberries, blackberries can be used – sprinkle a little sugar over the frozen fruit to sweeten it.
- You can miss out the spice from the filling or you could add it to the crumble topping.

Fruity Brioche Bread and Butter Pudding

Ingredients:

Butter (softened) · 15g (1 dessertspoon)
Brioche (sliced) · 120g (4 slices)
Raspberries · 75g mashed with 15ml (1 level tablespoon) caster sugar
Cream (double) · 150ml carton
Milk · 45mls (3 tablespoons)
Eggs · 1
Caster Sugar · 25g (1 tablespoon)
Vanilla Extract/Essence · 2.5mls (½ teaspoon)
Ground Nutmeg or Cinnamon · 2.5mls (½ teaspoon)
Butter for greasing

Method:

1. Set oven to Gas Mark 4, 180°C.

2. Grease an ovenproof dish.

3. Butter one side of each slice of the brioche and cut each slice into 4 triangles.

4. Place half of the brioche butter side up into the base of the greased oven proof dish overlapping slightly.

5. Spread the raspberries mashed with the sugar over the brioche.

6. Place the remaining brioche slices butter side up on the top of the raspberries.

7. Place the cream, milk, egg, 25g caster sugar, vanilla and nutmeg into a bowl and whisk together with a fork to mix.

8. Pour the mixture all over the brioche and leave to stand for 15 minutes – make sure the brioche is all covered by the milk mixture.

9. Bake for about 30 minutes until golden brown and there is no runny liquid in the middle.

Why Not Try: A tablespoon of sultanas can be used instead of the raspberries.

Panettone Bread and Butter Pudding

Ingredients:

Panettone · 250g (approx. 5 slices)
Butter (softened) · 25g (1 tablespoon)
Eggs · 2
Cream (double) · 150ml carton
Milk · 225mls
Vanilla Extract/Essence · 5ml (1 teaspoon)
Brown Sugar · 25g (1 tablespoon)
Butter for greasing

Method:

1. Set oven to Gas Mark 4, 180°C.

2. Grease an oven proof dish with a little of the butter for greasing.

3. Cut the panettone into wedges – leave the crusts on.

4. Spread the slices with the softened butter and cut or tear into smaller pieces and place in the dish butter side up

5. Whisk the eggs, cream, milk, vanilla essence/extract and half the brown sugar together.

6. Pour the egg mixture over the panettone and leave to sit for 20 minutes.

7. Sprinkle the rest of the sugar on the top and place in the oven for about 25-30 minutes until it is golden brown and set

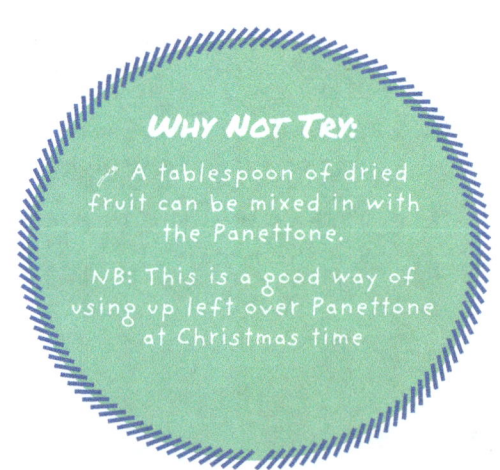

Why Not Try:
A tablespoon of dried fruit can be mixed in with the Panettone.

NB: This is a good way of using up left over Panettone at Christmas time

Summer Fruit Brulee

Ingredients:

Summer Fruits (fresh or defrosted if frozen) · 250g
Maple Syrup or Runny Honey · 1 tablespoon
Cream (double) · 150ml carton
Natural Yoghurt · 150ml carton
Soft Brown Sugar (dark) · 25g
Caster Sugar · 25g (1 tablespoon)

Method:

1. Place the summer fruits in a bowl, pour over the maple syrup or honey and leave to stand for 10 minutes.

2. Place the summer fruits into a small heat proof dish, or heat proof ramekin dishes.

3. Whisk the double cream until it forms soft peaks.

4. Fold the yoghurt into the cream.

5. Spread the yoghurt and cream mixture over the fruit and place in the refrigerator.

6. Heat the grill so that it is really hot for caramelising the sugar.

7. Mix the soft brown and caster sugars together and sprinkle evenly and thickly over the cream mixture.

8. Place the dish under the hot grill until the sugar is caramelised (if you have a cook's blow torch then this can also be used to brown the sugars very quickly).

9. Refrigerate until needed (putting the Brulee in the fridge will ensure a crunchy topping).

Why Not Try:

Use a 300ml carton of Crème Fraiche instead of the cream and natural yoghurt.

Fruit Sponge Pudding

Ingredients:

Base:
Cooking Apples / Rhubarb · 250g
Granulated Sugar · 50g

} 250g frozen fruit (eg pineapples, peaches)
250g tinned fruit in natural juice

Sponge:
Self-Raising Flour · 75g
Caster Sugar · 50g
Margarine · 50g
Eggs · 1 at room temperature
Water (warm) · 15ml (1 tablespoon)

Method:

1. Set oven to Gas Mark 5, 190°C.

2. Wash fruit if using fresh. Peel, core and slice apples or slice rhubarb thinly.

3. Place in a pan with 2 x 15 ml water and the 50g granulated sugar.

4. Stew gently with the lid on for about 5 minutes until soft. Place in oven proof dish

5. If using tinned fruit, cut into smaller pieces if required. If using frozen fruit place in an ovenproof dish (no need to defrost it)

6. Place all the ingredients for the sponge into a baking bowl and beat together with a wooden spoon or an electric mixer until smooth and creamy.

7. Carefully spread sponge mixture over the top of the fruit.

Bake for about 25 minutes until golden brown and firm to touch.

Strawberry and Almond Crumble

Ingredients:

Base:
Strawberries (fresh or frozen) · 250g
Caster Sugar · 25g
Ground Almonds · 10ml (2 teaspoons)
Vanilla Extract/Essence · 10mls (2 teaspoons)

Crumble Topping:
Plain Flour · 100g (4 tablespoons)
Ground Almonds · 25g (1 tablespoon)
Margarine or Butter · 50g
Flaked Almonds · 50g (4 tablespoons)
Soft Brown Sugar · 25g (1 tablespoon)

Method:

1. Set oven to Gas Mark 6, 200°C.

2. Prepare the base:
   - Wash and dry strawberries
   - Cut the strawberries into slices.
   - In a bowl mix the strawberries, ground almonds, caster sugar and vanilla.
   - Place into an oven proof dish.

3. Prepare the topping:
   - Place the flour into a large bowl.
   - Add the margarine to the bowl and rub in with the fingers until the mixture resembles fine breadcrumbs (you can use a food processor for this)

4. Stir in the ground almonds, flaked almonds and the soft brown sugar.

5. Spoon the topping over the strawberries then place in the oven to bake.

6. Bake for about 20 minutes until golden brown.

Why Not Try:

- The strawberries can be changed to raspberries or blackberries.
- To make it a bit easier use 4 tablespoons of ready prepared crumble mix and stir the ground almonds etc into it.

NB: If the strawberries have gone a little soft this is a good way of using them up.

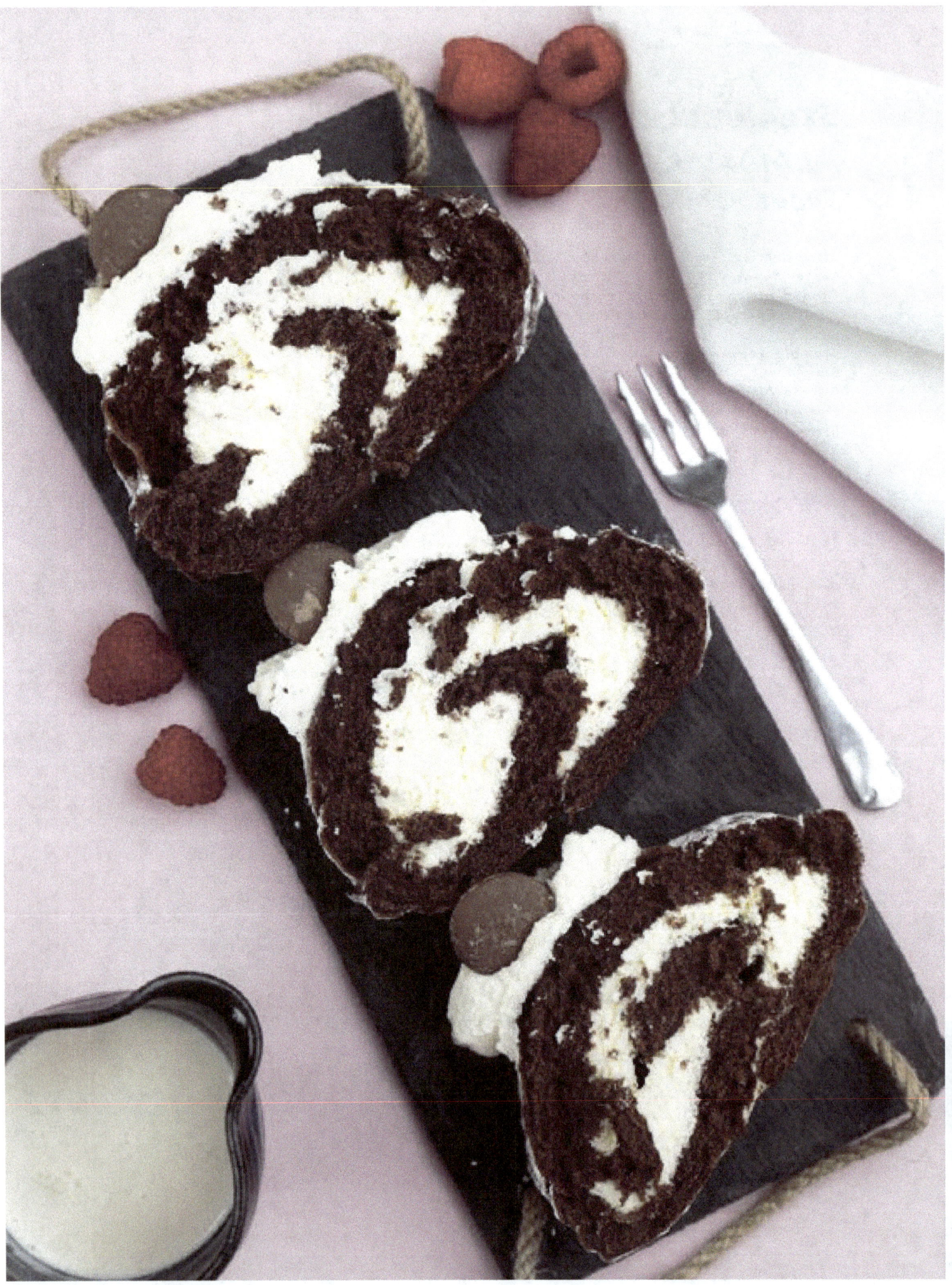

Chocolate Roulade

Ingredients:

Cake:
Drinking Chocolate · 1 level tablespoon

Plain Flour · 50g
Cocoa · 25g
Caster sugar · 75g
Eggs · 3 at room temperature

Filling:
Cream (double) · 150ml carton

Method:

1. Set oven to Gas Mark 7, 220°C.
2. Grease and line a Swiss roll tin with greaseproof paper (see Kitchen Journal)
3. Sieve the flour and drinking chocolate on to a plate.
4. Whisk eggs and sugar in a bowl until thick and creamy (the mixture should resemble whipped cream)
5. Carefully fold the sieved flour and chocolate powder into the egg mixture.
6. Turn the mixture into the greased tin and bake for 8-10 minutes.
7. Place a clean piece of greaseproof paper onto a clear work space and sprinkle with caster sugar.
8. Remove the sponge from the oven and turn upside down on to the sugared paper.
9. Remove the Swiss roll tin and carefully peel the greaseproof paper off in strips, taking care not to tear the sponge.
10. Trim the crisp edges with a sharp knife.
11. Turn in the edge neatly and roll up the sponge with a fresh piece of greaseproof paper inside.
12. Place on a cooling tray and set aside to cool.
13. Whisk the cream to soft peak consistency.
14. Unroll the cold Swiss roll, remove the paper and spread with the cream.
15. Carefully re-roll, making sure the cream doesn't ooze out of the sides.
16. Dust the surface with icing sugar.

Apples Stuffed with Raspberries

Ingredients:

Eating Apple (skin on) · 1
Raspberries (fresh or frozen) · 75g (3 tablespoons)
Maple Syrup · 15ml (1 tablespoon)

Method:

1. Set oven to Gas Mark 6, 200°C.
2. Wash the apple and remove the core.
3. Cut a slit round the apple skin to prevent it bursting.
4. Place the apple into an oven proof dish.
5. Fill the centre of the apple with the raspberries, pressing them in firmly.
6. Spoon the maple syrup over the top of the raspberries.
7. Cover with tin foil if and bake in the oven for about 20 minutes until soft when pierced with a knife.

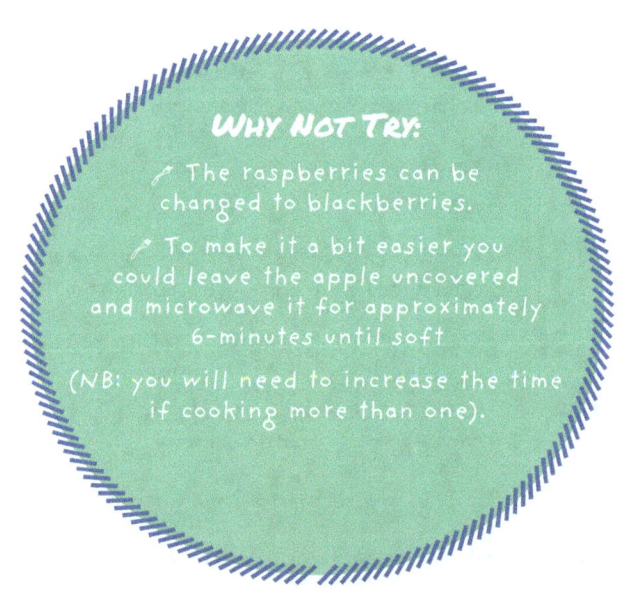

Why Not Try:

- The raspberries can be changed to blackberries.
- To make it a bit easier you could leave the apple uncovered and microwave it for approximately 6-minutes until soft

(NB: you will need to increase the time if cooking more than one).

Poached Pears with Chocolate Sauce

Ingredients:

Pears:
Pears (eating and fairly hard) - 4
Caster Sugar - 50g (2 tablespoons)
Water - 300mls

Chocolate Sauce:
Caster Sugar - 75g
Soft Brown Sugar - 75g
Cocoa/Drinking Chocolate - 75g
Milk - 100mls
Vanilla Essence/Extract - 5mls (1 teaspoon)
Butter - 25g

Method:

1. Place the 300mls of water in a pan with the caster sugar and bring to the boil
2. Peel the pears using a peeler.
3. Cut pears into quarters (lengthwise) and remove the core with a sharp knife.
4. Place the quarters into the syrup and simmer gently with the lid on for about 10 minutes until tender.
5. Remove from the heat and allow to cool in the liquid.

   Chocolate Sauce:

6. Put all the ingredients for the chocolate sauce into a pan.
7. Stir over a low heat until the sugars have dissolved.
8. Slowly bring to the boil and boil briskly without stirring for 2 minutes or until the sauce coats the back of the spoon.

   (NB: If a more fudge-like sauce is preferred, boil sauce for an extra 2-3 minutes)

Why Not Try:

Try with a Raspberry Coulis:
Raspberries (fresh or frozen) - 100g (4 tablespoons) Icing Sugar - 25g (1 tablespoon)

1. Place the raspberries and icing sugar into a jug.
2. Blend using a hand blender or potato masher/fork until smooth.

(NB: Strain the raspberry puree through a sieve to remove the seeds).

Mix and Match Cheesecake

Ingredients:

Base:
Digestive Biscuits · 100g (see chart below)
Margarine · 50g

Filling:
Cream Cheese · 75g
Caster Sugar · 50g
Yoghurt (thick set) · 1 small carton (see chart below)
Cream (double) · 150ml carton

Method:

1. Crush biscuits in a plastic bag or food processor.
2. Melt margarine in a pan then add crushed biscuits.
3. Press mixture into base of lightly greased sandwich tin with a metal spoon.
4. Place cream cheese and sugar for the filling into a large bowl and cream together until smooth.
5. Mix in the yoghurt to cream cheese and sugar.
6. Whip up cream in a separate bowl (do not over whip as it will turn to butter).
7. Carefully fold in one rounded tablespoonful of cream to yoghurt mixture.
8. Pour mixture over biscuit base and place in fridge to set.
9. Place remainder of cream into a piping bag (optional).
10. When set decorate cheesecake with cream and fruit.

Mix and Match Cheesecake

Decoration
Select your **topping**

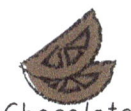
Chocolate Orange

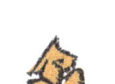
Honeycomb pieces

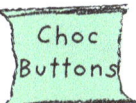
Choc Buttons

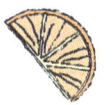
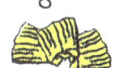
Grated Chocolate

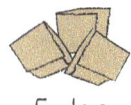
Mandarin segments

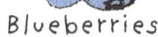
Pineapple

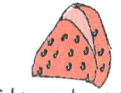
Fudge pieces

Blueberries

Strawberries

Raspberries

Filling
Select your **yoghurt**

Strawberry

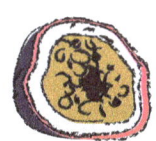
Passionfruit

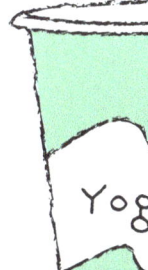
Lemon

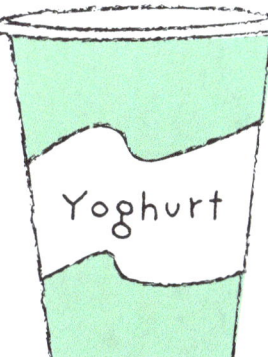
Yoghurt

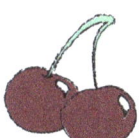
Black Cherry

Hazelnut

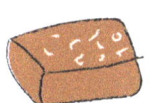
Salted Caramel

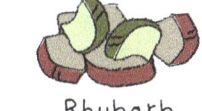
Rhubarb

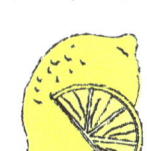
Fudge

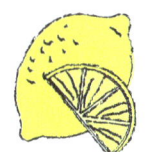

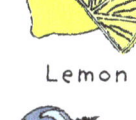
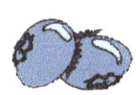
Raspberry

Blueberry

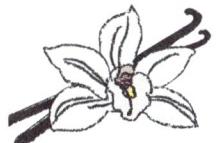
Vanilla

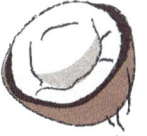
Coconut

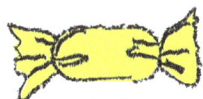
Toffee

Base
Select your **biscuit**

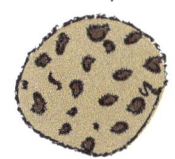
Chocolate Chip Cookies

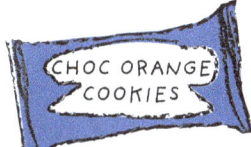
CHOC ORANGE COOKIES

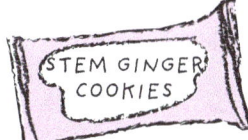
STEM GINGER COOKIES

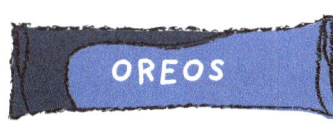
OREOS

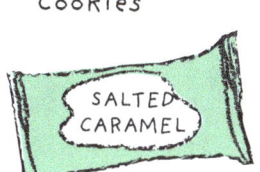
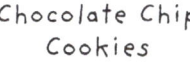
SALTED CARAMEL

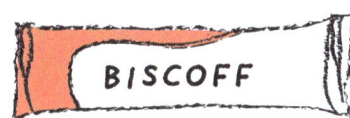
BISCOFF

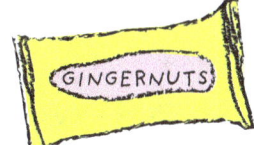
GINGERNUTS

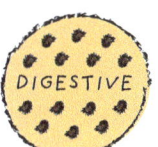
DIGESTIVE

Pecan, Maple, & Vanilla Cheesecake

Ingredients:

Pecan Shortbread:
Butter (softened) · 100g
Plain Flour · 100g
Icing Sugar · 50g
Cornflour · 50g
Pecan Nuts (crushed) · 50g
Maple Syrup · 10mls (2 teaspoons)

Cheesecake Base:
Butter · 100g
Pecan Shortbread Biscuits from recipe above (crushed)

Filling:
Cream (double) · 300ml carton
Greek Yoghurt · 200mls
Lemon · 1 (Zest)
Vanilla Extract/Essence · 5mls (1 teaspoon)
Icing Sugar · 50g (2 tablespoons)

Decoration:
Strawberries

Method:

1. Set oven to Gas Mark 4, 170°C.
2. Place all ingredients for shortbread in a food processor and mix together on high speed to form a dough.
3. Cut the dough into 8 pieces, flatten and place on baking tray and bake place in the oven for 10 - 15 minutes until it starts to turn golden brown.
4. Once cooked remove from oven and cool on the baking tray.
5. Crush the shortbread biscuits in a plastic bag.
6. Melt the butter for the base in a pan and add the crushed biscuits.
7. Place base mix into a sandwich tin or flan dish and press down with the back of a spoon.
8. Whisk cream to a soft peak consistency, then grate the zest of the lemon.
9. Mix yoghurt, icing sugar, lemon zest and vanilla extract together and fold in the whipped cream.
10. Spoon this mixture over the base and place in the fridge to set.

White Chocolate & Jamaican Rum Cheesecake

Ingredients:

Ginger Nut or 'Biscoff' / 'Biscotti' biscuits (crushed) · 100g
Butter · 50g
Rum (Jamaican) · 15mls (1 tablespoon)
Cream Cheese · 100g
Caster Sugar · 25g (1 tablespoon)
Cream (double) · 300ml carton

Cooking Chocolate (white) · 75g

Method:

1. Melt the butter in a pan then add the biscuits and mix.
2. Turn biscuit mixture into a small sandwich tin and press down with the back of a metal spoon. Put in the fridge to chill.
3. Beat the cream cheese with the caster sugar.
4. Whisk the cream until soft peak consistency.
5. Melt the chocolate over a pan of hot water or in the microwave.
6. Mix the cream cheese with the rum and mix with the melted chocolate.
7. Fold 2/3 of the whipped cream into the cream cheese and chocolate mixture.
8. Spoon this topping over the biscuit base and chill.
9. Decorate with the rest of the cream.

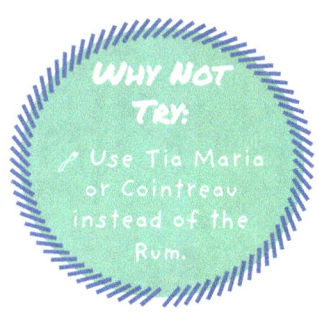

Why Not Try:
Use Tia Maria or Cointreau instead of the Rum.

Sweet Treats

Crunchy Biscuits

Ingredients:

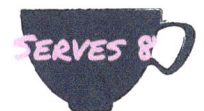 Serves 8

- Margarine (soft) • 50g
- Caster Sugar • 36g
- Self-Raising flour • 50g
- Porridge Oats • 50g
- Syrup • 2.5mls
- Boiling Water • 5mls

Method:

1. Set oven to Gas Mark 4, 180°C.
2. Cream margarine and sugar together until soft and well mixed.
3. Measure the flour and porridge oats on to a plate.
4. Dissolve syrup in a cup with the boiling water.
5. Stir the syrup mixture into the margarine and sugar.
6. Gradually mix in the flour and oats to make a firm dough (you may need to bring the mixture together by hand).
7. Divide the dough into 8 even pieces.
8. Roll each piece into a ball and place on a greased baking tray.
9. Flatten each biscuit with the back of a fork dipped in a little flour.
10. Place into the oven and bake for approximately 15 minutes until golden brown.
11. Leave biscuits to cool on baking tray for a few minutes to allow them to set then remove to a cooling tray.

Oat and Sultana Cookies

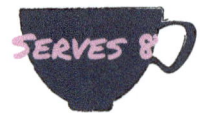

Serves 8

Ingredients:

Margarine (soft) • 50g
Caster Sugar • 100g
Egg • 1
Plain flour • 50g
Salt • pinch
Baking Powder • 1.25mls (¼ teaspoon)
Porridge Oats • 50g
Sultanas • 50g
Sesame Seeds • 10mls (2 teaspoons) (optional)

Method:

1. Set oven to Gas Mark 4, 180°C.
2. Lightly grease a baking tray.
3. Cream the sugar and margarine in a large bowl or mixer until light and fluffy.
4. Gradually add beaten egg and beat well until smooth.
5. Add the flour, salt, and baking powder to the bowl and mix well.
6. Add the porridge oats, sultanas and sesame seeds and mix thoroughly together.
7. Place 8 teaspoonfuls of mixture well apart on the greased baking tray and flatten slightly with the back of a fork. (Tip — dip the fork in a little flour to stop it sticking).
8. Bake in the oven for 15 minutes or until golden brown.
9. Leave the biscuits to cool slightly on the baking tray before transferring them to a cooling tray.

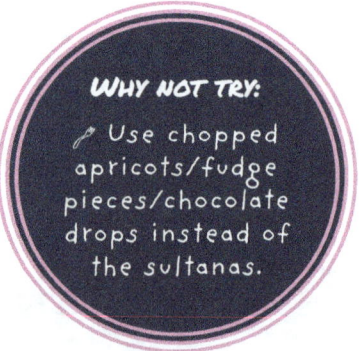

Why not try:
Use chopped apricots/fudge pieces/chocolate drops instead of the sultanas.

Shortbread Biscuits

Ingredients:

Butter (slightly salted) • 200g (softened)
Plain flour • 200g
Cornflour • 100g
Icing Sugar • 100g
(For Highlander Biscuits add **Demerara Sugar** • 50g)

Method:

1. Set oven to Gas Mark 4, 180°C
2. Carefully measure out ingredients using scales (NB: it is important to accurately weigh the ingredients for this recipe).
3. Cut up the butter/margarine into smaller pieces.
4. Place all ingredients into a food processor and mix on high speed until mixture forms a dough.
5. Carefully remove from processor and place on to a lightly floured work surface.
6. Roll out to 1cm thickness and cut out biscuits using a cutter.
7. Place on a baking tray and mark the surface with a fork.
8. Bake in oven for 10-15 minutes or until golden brown (NB: the biscuits will be soft to touch when they come out of the oven as they will set when cool).
9. Sprinkle with caster sugar and allow to cool on the baking tray before removing to cooling tray.

Highlander Biscuits

Method:

1. Make a batch of shortbread as per the recipe above.
2. Remove mixture from the bowl, divide into two and shape into a sausage shape (you can use a little flour on the work surface to prevent it sticking).
3. Place the Demerara sugar on to a piece of greaseproof paper
4. Roll the shortbread in the sugar then slice into even sized biscuits (about 1cm thick).
5. Place flat side down on the baking tray and bake for 10-15 minutes or until golden brown
6. Remove tray from oven and leave biscuits on the tray to cool slightly before transferring to a cooling tray.

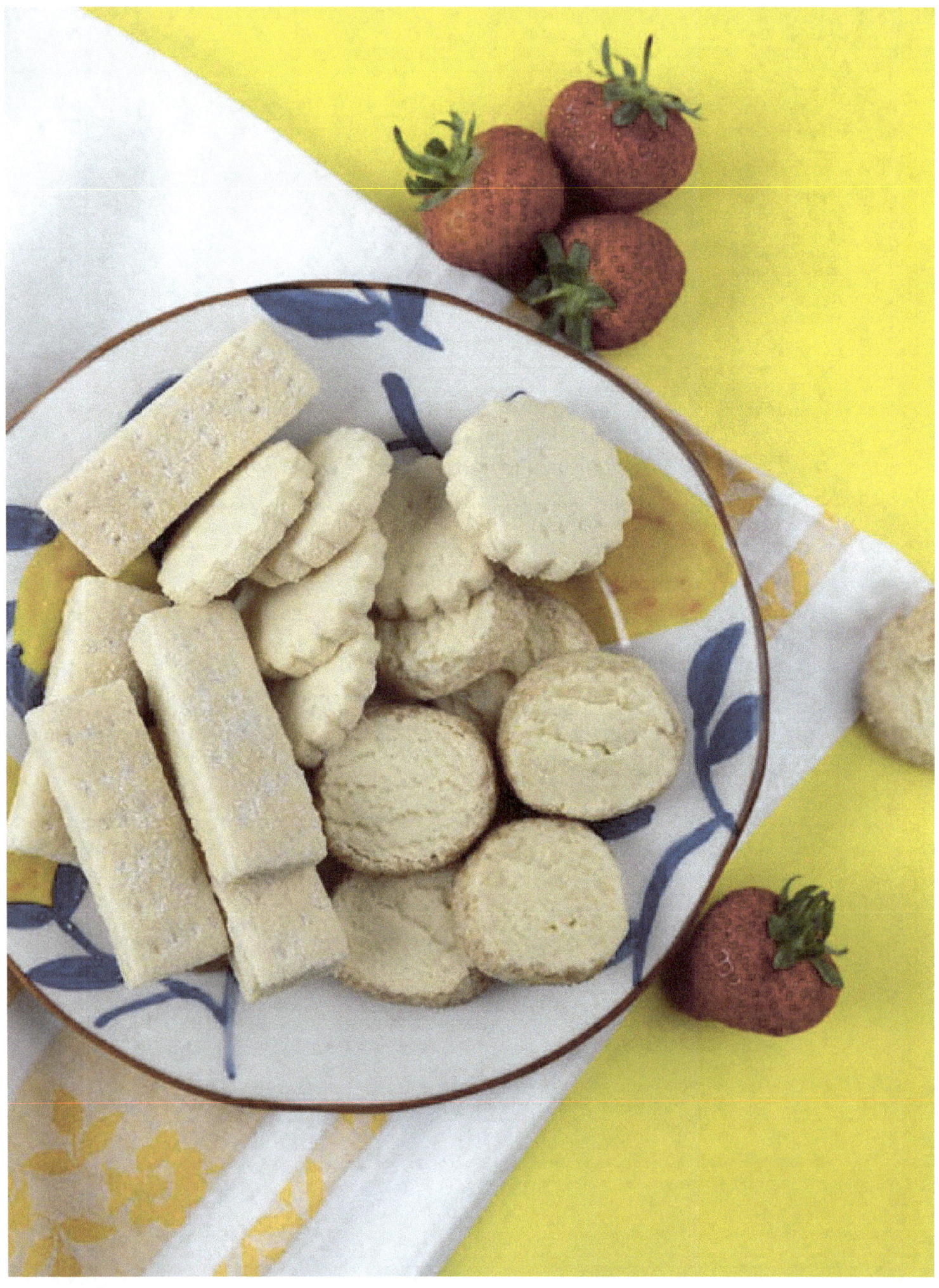

Dippy-Dunk Cookies

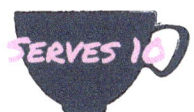

Serves 10

Ingredients:

Cookies:
Margarine (soft) • 50g
Caster Sugar • 100g
Egg • 1
Plain flour • 50g
Salt • pinch
Baking Powder • 1.25mls (¼ teaspoon)
Porridge Oats • 50g
Fruit Flakes • 1 small packet

Dip:
Fruit Yoghurt (thick set) • 1 small carton
Fruit Flakes • 1 small packet

Why not try:
- Use chopped apricots/fudge pieces/chocolate drops instead of the fruit flakes.
- Stir 2 teaspoons of jam into the yoghurt dip.
- Use a chocolate mousse instead of yoghurt and add some Chocolate Drops/Smarties instead of fruit flakes.

Method:

1. Set oven to Gas Mark 4, 180°C.
2. Lightly grease a baking tray.
3. Cream the sugar and margarine in a large bowl or mixer until light and fluffy.
4. Gradually add beaten egg and beat well until smooth.
5. Add the flour, salt and baking powder to the bowl and mix well.
6. Add the porridge oats and fruit flakes and mix thoroughly together.
7. Place the mixture on to a very lightly floured work surface and shape and flatten into a rectangle (approximately 8cm by 20 cm).
8. Cut the mixture into 10 small rectangular cookies (approximately 2cm by 8cm)
9. Bake in the oven for 15 minutes or until golden brown.
10. Leave the biscuits to cool slightly on the baking tray before transferring them to a cooling tray.
11. For the dip, mix the fruit flakes into the yoghurt.

Valentine's Biscuits

Ingredients:

Biscuits:
Margarine • 75g
Self-Raising Flour • 100g
Caster Sugar • 50g
Egg • 1 (beaten)

Filling:
Jam • 1 to 2 tablespoons

Topping:
Icing sugar • 1 tablespoon

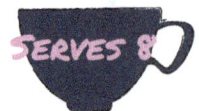

Serves 8

Method:

1. Set oven to Gas Mark 4, 180°C.
2. Grease 2 baking trays.
3. Place flour and margarine into bowl and rub in until mixture resembles fine breadcrumbs (this can be done in a food processor).
4. Stir in the sugar.
5. Add the beaten egg a little at a time until mixture comes together.
6. Turn out on to a lightly floured work surface and knead gently until smooth.
7. Roll out to ½ cm thickness, pierce with a fork then cut out using a loveheart shaped cutter.
8. Place biscuits on a baking tray and bake for 12-15 minutes or until golden brown.
9. Leave biscuits on baking tray to cool slightly then transfer to a cooling tray.
10. When cold sandwich the biscuits together with jam.
11. Dust the tops of the biscuits with icing sugar.

Why not try:

- Cut out a smaller heart in the centre of half of the biscuits so you can see the jam when sandwiched together.
- Spread a layer of butter icing under the jam before sandwiching them together.

Truffles

Ingredients:

Margarine (soft) • 25g
Drinking Chocolate • 25g (1 tablespoon) NB: if using cocoa powder use half the amount as it is a strong flavour)
Coconut • 25g (1 tablespoon)
Digestive Biscuits (crushed) • 100g
Condensed Milk • 3 tablespoons (approx)

Method:

1. Cream margarine and chocolate powder in large bowl or food processor.
2. Add coconut, digestive biscuits and condensed milk to bowl.
3. Mix to a soft but not too sticky mixture.
4. Take a teaspoonful of mixture and shape into a ball.
5. Roll in coconut or chocolate powder.

Halloween Truffles

Ingredients:

Coconut • 50g (2 tablespoons)
Orange Food Colouring • A few drops
Writing Icing Tube • 1 Black / Chocolate

Method:

1. Colour the coconut by stirring in the orange food colouring with a fork.
2. Roll the shaped truffles in the orange coloured coconut.
3. Use black / chocolate icing to decorate with eyes and nose etc.
4. End results should resemble a pumpkin.

> **Cook's Tip**
> If having difficulty shaping the truffles, flatten the mixture into a tin lined with clingfilm, sprinkle the coconut/drinking chocolate lightly over the top and place in the fridge to set. Once set remove from the tin and cut into small squares.

Malteser Slice

Ingredients:

Base:
Cooking Chocolate (milk) • 200g
Margarine • 100g
Syrup • 3 tablespoons
Digestive Biscuits • 200g

Topping:
Cooking Chocolate (milk) • 100g
Maltesers • 1 large bag

Method:

1. Crush biscuits either in the food processor or in a food bag with a rolling pin.

2. Gently melt the chocolate, margarine and syrup in a pan. Do not boil.

3. Mix in the crushed digestive biscuits.

4. Turn the mixture into a cake tin and press down with the back of a metal spoon (the mixture will look sloppy at this stage but will set).

5. Melt the chocolate for the topping in either a bowl over a pan of hot water or in the microwave.

6. Pour the melted chocolate over the surface of the biscuit mixture and smooth.

7. Place the Maltesers over the surface (space out).

8. Allow mixture to set at room temperature.

Why Not Try:

- Add a couple of tablespoons of sultanas to the biscuit mixture Use white chocolate or flavoured chocolate for the topping instead of milk chocolate.
- Use Hob Nob biscuits for an added texture and flavour.
- Use white or flavoured Maltesers.
- Alternatives to Maltesers that can be used are M&Ms, Smarties, Revels, Minstrels.

Cook's Tip

- Press the Maltesers into the biscuit mixture before covering with melted chocolate or carefully mix the Maltesers into the biscuit mixture before turning into the tin then coat with melted chocolate.

Bakewell Tart

Ingredients:

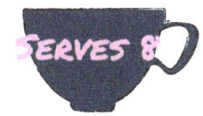
Serves 8

Pastry:
Ready Rolled Shortcrust/Sweet Shortcrust • 1 packet fresh pastry or 1 sweet pastry case already baked

Filling:
Jam • 2 tablespoons (own choice)

Sponge:
Margarine (soft) • 100g
Caster sugar • 100g
Self-Raising Flour • 100g
Eggs • 2 at room temperature
Water (warm) • 1 dessertspoon

> **WHY NOT TRY:**
> Use lemon curd or fruit pie filling instead of the jam.
> NB: You can use a flan dish instead of a sandwich tin for this recipe.

Serving Suggestion:

Cut into wedges to serve. Can be eaten warm and cold.
Serve a warm wedge on a plate with some ice cream and / or whipped cream for a dessert.

Method:

1. Set oven to Gas Mark 4, 180°C.
2. Unroll fresh pastry sheet and use to line a 20cm sandwich tin.
3. Spread jam over the base of the pastry case.
4. Place all the ingredients for the sponge into a large bowl and beat with an electric whisk until mixture is smooth and creamy.
5. Carefully spread sponge mixture over jam.
6. Place in oven and bake for 20 minutes approximately until golden brown and sponge springs back when touched.
7. Allow to cool slightly then dust lightly with icing sugar.

Mix and Match Sponge Cakes

Basic 'All-In-One' Sponge Mix

Ingredients:

Margarine (soft) • 100g
Caster Sugar • 100g
Self-Raising flour • 100g
Eggs • 2 at room temperature
Warm Water • 1 dessertspoon

Method:

1. Set oven to Gas Mark 4, 180°C.

2. Place all ingredients for cakes into a large bowl and beat using an electric mixer on high speed until light and fluffy.

3. Bake for 20 minutes approx. or until golden and springs back when pressed.

Basic Fatless Sponge Mix

Ingredients:

Caster Sugar • 50g
Self-Raising Flour • 50g
Eggs • 2 at room temperature

Method:

1. Set oven to Gas Mark 4, 180°C.

2. Sieve flour on to a plate.

3. Whisk eggs and sugar in a bowl until light and fluffy (the mixture should look like whipped cream).

4. Carefully fold in the sieved flour.

5. Bake for 10 to 15 minutes until golden brown and springs back when pressed.

Monster Cakes

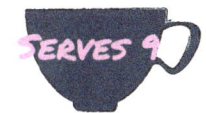

Serves 9

Ingredients:

Cakes:
Margarine or Butter (softened) • 100g
Self-Raising Flour • 100g
Caster Sugar • 100g
Eggs • 2 at room temperature

Decoration:
Margarine (soft) • 100g
Icing Sugar • 150g   } OR   buy a tub of ready-made icing
Vanilla Essence • 1.25mls (¼ teaspoon)

Coconut • 3 tablespoons
Food Colouring • A few drops
Mini Choc Chip Cookies • 1 small packet
Ready Roll White Icing • (small ball) OR 1 small packet white chocolate buttons
Ready Roll Black Icing • (small ball) OR Black / chocolate tube of writing icing

Method:

1. Set oven to Gas Mark 4, 180°C.
2. Place 9 paper cases in a patty/bun tin.
3. Place all ingredients for cakes into a large bowl and beat using an electric mixer on high speed until light and fluffy.
4. Divide mixture (using a dessertspoon) evenly between the nine paper cases.
5. Bake for approximately 15 – 20 minutes until golden brown and spring back when touched.
6. Remove from cake tins and place on a wire rack to cool.

Let's Decorate:

1. Make up the butter icing by placing the margarine in a bowl with the vanilla essence and beating in the icing sugar a spoonful at a time (you can make this in a food processor by adding all the ingredients together and mixing on a high speed until smooth).
2. Colour the coconut by stirring in the orange food colouring with a fork.
3. Spread butter icing on to each cake and then coat in the coloured coconut
4. Decorate with cookies to make cookie monsters
5. Make eyes from the ready roll icing.

Individual Sponge Cakes

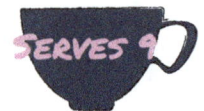 Serves 9

Ingredients:

Margarine or Butter (softened) • 100g
Self-Raising Flour • 100g
Caster Sugar • 100g
Eggs • 2 at room temperature

Method:

1. Set oven to Gas Mark 4, 180°C.
2. Place 9 paper cases in a patty/bun tin.
3. Place all ingredients for cakes into a large bowl and beat using an electric mixer on high speed until light and fluffy.
4. Divide mixture (using a dessertspoon) evenly between the nine paper cases.
5. Bake for approximately 15 – 20 minutes until golden brown and spring back when touched.
6. Remove from cake tins and allow to cool slightly.
7. Place cakes on a wire rack.
8. Dust with icing sugar when cool.

Why not try:
Add a tablespoon of sultanas/fruit flakes to the mixture before baking or place a teaspoon of sultanas/fruit flakes into the base of each paper case before spooning the mixture over the top of them.

Decorate the tops with some glace or butter icing once cold

Butterfly Cake

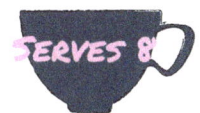

Ingredients:

Cakes:
Basic All in One Sponge Cake Mix • 1 batch (see recipe)

Filling:
Jam (own choice) • 2 tablespoons

Topping:
Icing Sugar • 100g
Cold water to mix (2-3 teaspoons)
Food colouring • a few drops (optional)

Decoration:
Smarties or Jelly Tots
Small chocolate flake

Method:

1. Set oven to Gas Mark 4, 180°C.

2. Grease and line two small round (15cm) sandwich/cake tins with greaseproof paper.

3. Place all the ingredients for the cakes into a large bowl and beat using an electric mixer on high speed until light and fluffy.

4. Divide mixture evenly between the two tins and smooth out the surface.

5. Bake for 20-25 minutes until golden brown and spring back when touched.

6. Remove from the oven, allow to cool slightly then run a knife round the edge of the cake tins and turn on to a cooling tray.

7. Peel off the greaseproof paper and set to one side to cool.

8. Sandwich the cold cakes together with jam.

9. Cut the cake in two and place on plate back to back (see diagram above).

10. Make up the glace icing (add the water a spoon at a time as too much water will make it too runny) and spread carefully over the wings of the butterfly.

11. Decorate the wings with the sweeties and place a small chocolate flake in centre of the cake.

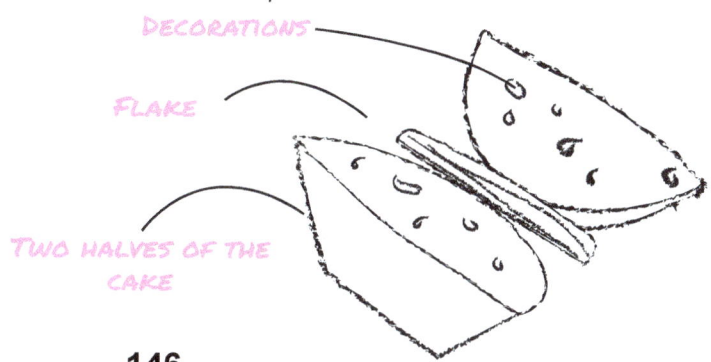

Chocolate Butterfly Cakes

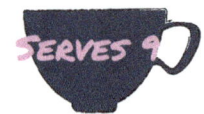
Serves 9

Ingredients:

Cakes:
Margarine (soft) • 100g
Caster Sugar • 100g
Self-Raising flour • 75g
Drinking Chocolate • 25g (if using Cocoa use slightly less as it is a rich flavour)
Eggs • 2 at room temperature
Warm Water • 1 dessertspoon

Topping:
Double Cream – 100mls
Mandarin Oranges (drained) – 9 (optional)

Method:

1. Set oven to Gas Mark 4, 180°C.
2. Place 9 paper cases into a patty/bun tin.
3. Place ingredients for cakes into a large bowl and beat with an electric mixer on high speed for 2-3 minutes until light and fluffy.
4. Divide mixture out evenly between paper cases.
5. Bake in oven for 20 minutes (approximately) or until cakes spring back when touched.
6. Remove from oven, transfer on to a cooling tray and allow to cool.
7. Whip cream carefully until thick (do not over whip as mixture will turn to butter).
8. Slice tops off cakes and place to one side.
9. Divide cream equally between cakes (either spoon it on or use a piping bag).
10. Split each lid in two and set back into tops of cakes to resemble wings.
11. Decorate each cake with a mandarin orange (optional).

> **Why not try:**
> Use butter icing instead of the fresh cream and use chocolate buttons/chips/sprinkles instead of the mandarin oranges.
>
> Cakes must be stored in a refrigerator and consumed within 24 hours unless the fresh cream and mandarin is replaced with butter icing.

Jammy Layer Cake

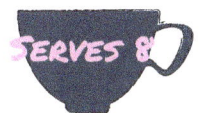
Serves 8

Ingredients:

Sponge:
Basic Fatless Sponge Mix - 1 batch (see recipe)

Filling:
Jam (own choice) - 2 tablespoons

Topping
Caster sugar

Method:

1. Set oven to Gas Mark 5, 190°C.

2. Grease and line a Swiss roll tin with greaseproof paper.

3. Sieve flour on to a plate.

4. Whisk eggs and sugar in a bowl until light and fluffy (the mixture should look like whipped cream)

5. Carefully fold in the sieved flour.

6. Turn the mixture into the greased tin and bake for 10-15 minutes until golden brown and springs back when touched.

7. Place the jam in a cup and mix with a spoon to soften it and set to one side.

8. Remove the sponge from the oven, turn on to a cooling tray and carefully remove the greaseproof paper. Set to one side to cool.

9. Carefully trim the two short edges off the sponge and then cut it into three equal pieces.

10. Place one piece of the sponge on to a plate then spread half the jam over the surface.

11. Place a second piece of the cake on top of this and repeat with the rest of the yoghurt jam.

12. Place the third layer of the cake over the top of this and sieve a thin layer of caster sugar over the top.

Why not try:

Flavour the sponge by sieving ½ teaspoon of cinnamon or mixed spice with the flour and use a half a tin of apple pie filling instead of jam.

Make the sponge chocolate by replacing a dessertspoon of the flour with chocolate powder and fill with chocolate spread or chocolate spread mixed with some thick cream instead of jam.

Mini Apple Crumble Tarts

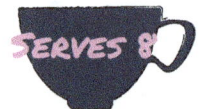
Serves 8

Ingredients:

Pastry / Topping:
Plain Flour · 75g
Wholemeal Flour · 75g
Margarine · 75g
Water (cold) · 4 teaspoons (approximately)
Soft Brown Sugar · 25g

Filling:
Apple Pie Filling · ½ tin

Serving Suggestions:

Serve hot or cold
Serve as a dessert with some ice-cream, fresh cream, custard or all three, or fromage frais for a healthier option.

Method:

1. Set oven to Gas Mark 6, 200°C.
2. Place flour into a large bowl, add margarine then rub in until it resembles fine breadcrumbs (this can be done in a food processor).
3. Remove 2 tablespoons of the mixture and place into a small bowl along with the brown sugar.
4. Set the small bowl to one side.
5. Carefully add cold water a teaspoonful at a time to the large bowl/food processor until mixture forms a stiff dough.
6. Turn dough out on to a lightly floured tabletop and knead lightly until smooth.
7. Roll out dough and cut out circles with a pastry cutter.
8. Place pastry circles into a patty tin (do not overstretch pastry)
9. Place a teaspoonful of pie filling into each pastry case.
10. Sprinkle a teaspoonful of the topping over the pie filling.
11. Bake for 10-15 minutes or until golden brown.

Mini Lemon Tarts

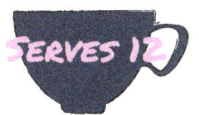 Serves 12

Ingredients:

Pastry:
Plain Flour · 100g
Margarine · 50g
Water (cold) · to mix

OR 1 packet fresh ready rolled Shortcrust pastry

Filling
Lemon Curd · 50g (2 tablespoons)

Decoration (optional):
Icing Sugar · to dust

Serving Suggestions:

Serve warm or cold
Serve as a dessert with some ice-cream, fresh cream, or creme fraiche for a healthier option.

Method:

1. Set oven to Gas Mark 4, 180°C.

   If making your own pastry:

2. Place plain flour for pastry into a large bowl or food processor.
3. Rub in the margarine until mixture resembles fine breadcrumbs.
4. Carefully add cold water a teaspoonful at a time to the large bowl/food processor until mixture forms a stiff dough.
5. Turn pastry out on to a floured work surface and knead lightly.
6. Roll pastry out and cut out thin circles using a pastry cutter and use to line a patty tin.
7. If using ready rolled pastry — cut out circles
8. Place ½ a teaspoon of lemon curd into each pastry case (do not overfill).
9. Place in oven and bake for 10-15 minutes until pastry is golden.
10. Allow to cool slightly then remove from patty tin.
11. Dust with icing sugar when cold.

Bonfire Cake

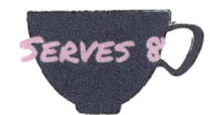
Serves 8

Ingredients:

Cakes:
Basic All in One Sponge Cake Mix • 1 batch (see recipe)

Filling and decorations:
1 tub butter icing
1 tablespoon jam
Selection of sweets
Chocolate flakes

Method:

1. Set oven to Gas Mark 4, 180°C.
2. Grease and line two small round sandwich/cake tins (15cm) with greaseproof paper.
3. Place all the ingredients for the cakes into a large bowl and beat using an electric mixer on high speed until light and fluffy.
4. Divide mixture evenly between the two tins and smooth out the surface.
5. Bake for 20-25 minutes until golden brown and spring back when touched.
6. Remove from the oven, allow to cool slightly then run a knife round the edge of the cake tins and turn cakes out on to a cooling tray.
7. Peel off the greaseproof paper and set to one side to cool.
8. Sandwich the cold cakes together with jam and a little butter icing.
9. Decorate top of cake using the butter icing, sweeties, flakes etc in the theme of a bonfire.

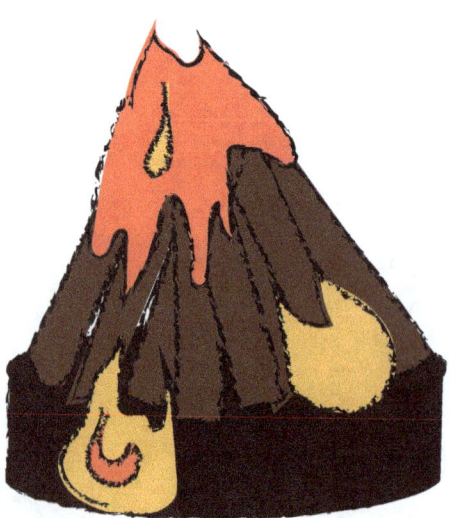

Why not try:
- Make it a Chocolate Bonfire Cake by changing the 100g of SR flour to 75g and adding 25g drinking chocolate.
- Use chocolate butter icing mixed with a little chocolate spread for the centre and top and decorate with some flakes and standing up to look like a bonfire and chocolate chips/sweets.

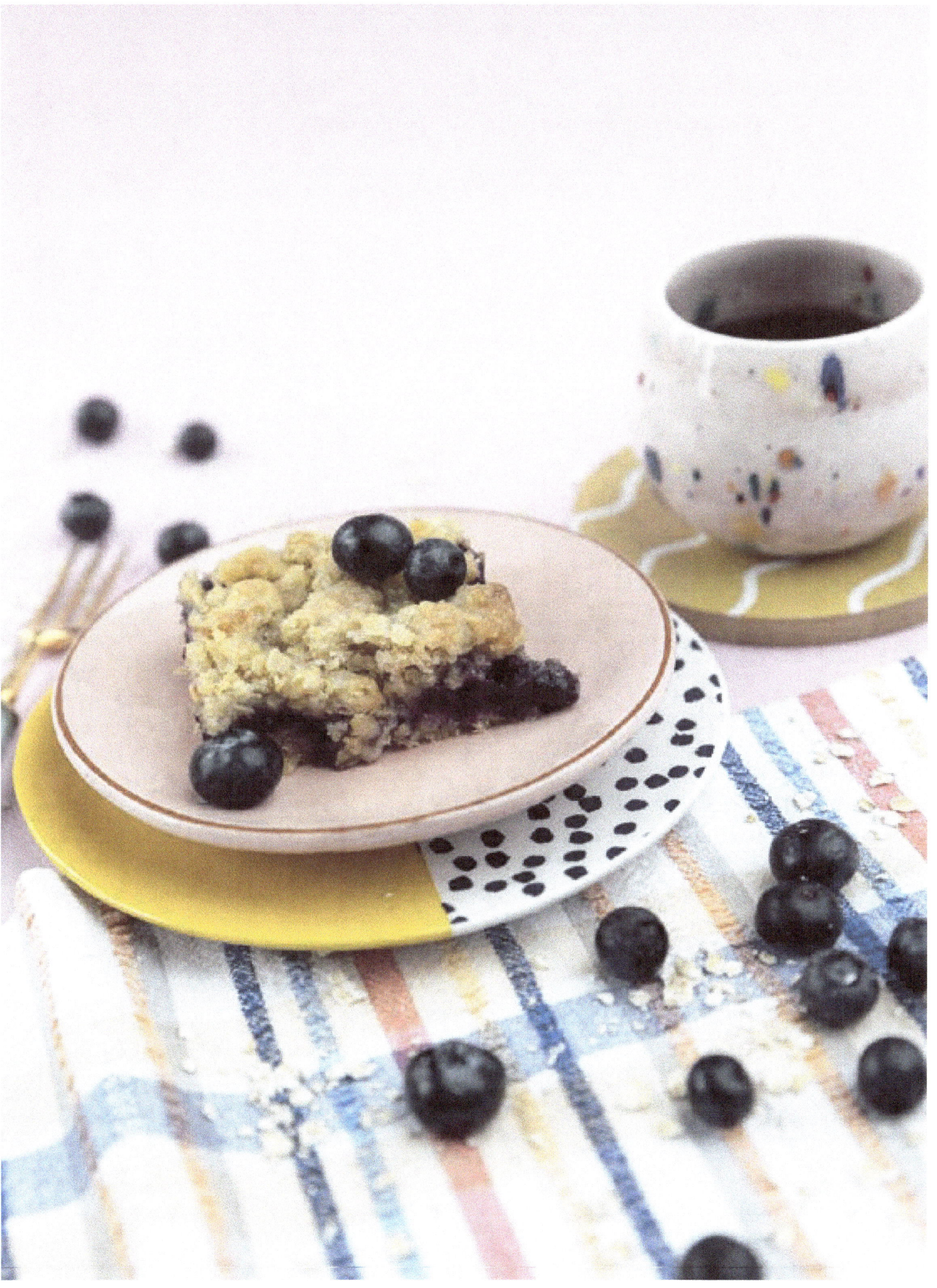

Blueberry Crumble Traybake

Ingredients:

Crumble Mix:
Plain Flour • 100g
Porridge Oats • 250g
Caster Sugar • 250g
Margarine or Butter • 200g
Cinnamon (ground) • 2.5ml (½ teaspoon)

Filling:
Blueberries • 300g
Caster Sugar • 100g
Cornflour • 30ml
Lemon • 1 to give 30mls lemon juice

Serving Suggestions:

This can also be served as a dessert with ice cream or crème fraîche.

> **Why not try:**
> - Use fresh raspberries or brambles instead of blueberries.
> - Try a mincemeat version for Christmas.

Method:

1. Set oven to Gas mark 5, 190°C.

2. Line a baking tray or foil tray bake of 30 x 20 cm (12 x 8 inches approx.) with non-stick baking paper.

3. For the filling place the blueberries, cornflour, 100g caster sugar and lemon juice in a pan. Bring to the boil, stirring all the time until the mixture has thickened — about 2 minutes.

4. For the crumble mix place the flour, porridge oats, 250g of caster sugar and the cinnamon. Into a baking bowl.

5. Add the margarine and rub in until the mixture looks like rough crumbs (this can be done in a food processor).

6. Place half of the crumb mixture in the baking tray and smooth over the base of the tray with the back of a metal spoon..

7. Carefully spread the blueberry mixture over the top of the crumble mixture.

8. Place the remaining crumble mixture evenly over the top of the blueberry mixture.

9. Bake for about 25 - 35 minutes until just browned. Leave to cool in the tray and then cut into squares/ bars.

Lemon Drizzle Cakes

Ingredients:

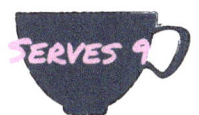 Serves 9

Margarine or Butter (softened) • 100g
Self-Raising Flour • 125g
Caster Sugar • 100g
Eggs • 2 at room temperature
Lemon Curd • 50g
Lemon (grated rind and juice) • 1

Topping:
Caster Sugar • 2 tablespoons
Lemon Juice • 1 tablespoon

Method:

1. Set oven to Gas Mark 5, 190°C.
2. Grease and line a loaf tin or place 9 paper cases into a patty tin.
3. Grate the rind of the lemon, cut the lemon in half and remove the juice. Set to one side.
4. Cream margarine and sugar in a large bowl until soft (use an electric whisk for this).
5. Beat eggs in a cup, sieve flour on to a plate and measure lemon curd into a small bowl.
6. Beat the flour and eggs into the creamed margarine and sugar mixture until smooth.
7. Beat in the lemon curd and lemon rind until well mixed.
8. Divide the mixture evenly between the 9 paper cases or place in the greased and lined loaf tin.
9. Bake in oven until the mixture springs back when touched and are golden brown (15-20 minutes for the individual cakes / 45 minutes if using the loaf tin).
10. Place the lemon juice and sugar for the topping in a cup and mix with a teaspoon.
11. Drizzle this lemon mixture over the warm cakes/loaf and allow to cool.

Mars Bar Traybake

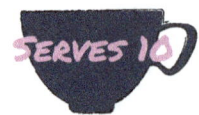
Serves 10

Ingredients:

Mars Bars • 5 standard-size (roughly cut or broken into pieces)
Butter • 150g
Rice Krispies to absorb the mixture • approx 100g
Syrup • 30ml (2 level tablespoons)
Milk Cooking Chocolate • 200g

Serving Suggestions:

Cut the set mixture out with animal etc cutters if serving to kids.

Method:

1. Use a baking tray or tin foil tray 30 x 20 cm (12 x 8 inches approx).
2. Melt the butter, syrup and Mars bars in a small pan or in a microwave.
3. When it's all melted, add the Rice Krispies and stir until they are all coated with the chocolate mixture.
4. Press the mixture into the lined tin and leave to set.
5. Melt the chocolate in either the microwave (stirring regularly) or in a bowl over a pan of hot water.
6. Pour the melted chocolate over the Rice Krispie mixture and smooth.
7. Cut into squares when cold.

Why not try:

Add some sultanas, smarties, chocolate chips to the mixture before turning into the tin (end of method 3)

NB: If you boil this mixture in method 2 the traybake will be very hard

Lemon Drizzle Cakes

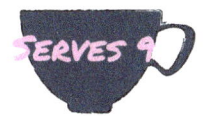

Serves 9

Ingredients:

Margarine or Butter (softened) • 100g
Self-Raising Flour • 125g
Caster Sugar • 100g
Eggs • 2 at room temperature
Lemon Curd • 50g
Lemon (grated rind and juice) • 1

Topping:
Caster Sugar • 2 tablespoons
Lemon Juice • 1 tablespoon

Method:

1. Set oven to Gas Mark 5, 190°C.
2. Grease and line a loaf tin or place 9 paper cases into a patty tin.
3. Grate the rind of the lemon, cut the lemon in half and remove the juice. Set to one side.
4. Cream margarine and sugar in a large bowl until soft (use an electric whisk for this).
5. Beat eggs in a cup, sieve flour on to a plate and measure lemon curd into a small bowl.
6. Beat the flour and eggs into the creamed margarine and sugar mixture until smooth.
7. Beat in the lemon curd and lemon rind until well mixed.
8. Divide the mixture evenly between the 9 paper cases or place in the greased and lined loaf tin.
9. Bake in oven until the mixture springs back when touched and are golden brown (15-20 minutes for the individual cakes / 45 minutes if using the loaf tin).
10. Place the lemon juice and sugar for the topping in a cup and mix with a teaspoon.
11. Drizzle this lemon mixture over the warm cakes/loaf and allow to cool.

Mars Bar Traybake

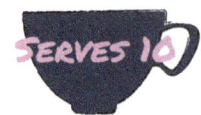
Serves 10

Ingredients:

Mars Bars • 5 standard-size (roughly cut or broken into pieces)
Butter • 150g
Rice Krispies to absorb the mixture • approx 100g
Syrup • 30ml (2 level tablespoons)
Milk Cooking Chocolate • 200g

Serving Suggestions:

Cut the set mixture out with animal etc cutters if serving to kids.

Method:

1. Use a baking tray or tin foil tray 30 x 20 cm (12 x 8 inches approx).
2. Melt the butter, syrup and Mars bars in a small pan or in a microwave.
3. When it's all melted, add the Rice Krispies and stir until they are all coated with the chocolate mixture.
4. Press the mixture into the lined tin and leave to set.
5. Melt the chocolate in either the microwave (stirring regularly) or in a bowl over a pan of hot water.
6. Pour the melted chocolate over the Rice Krispie mixture and smooth.
7. Cut into squares when cold.

Why not try:

Add some sultanas, smarties, chocolate chips to the mixture before turning into the tin (end of method 3)

NB: If you boil this mixture in method 2 the traybake will be very hard

Sticky Toffee Traybake

Ingredients:

Sponge:
Self-Raising Flour • 200g
Margarine or Butter (soft) • 175g
Dark Brown Sugar (soft) • 125g
Syrup • 150g
Treacle • 75g
Vanilla Extract/Essence • 5ml (1 teaspoon)
Eggs • 3 at room temperature
Double Cream • 30ml (2 tablespoons)

Fudge icing:
Margarine • 50g
Double Cream • 30ml (2 tablespoons)
Dark Brown Sugar (soft) • 75g
Icing Sugar • 40g

Method:

1. Set oven to Gas mark 4, 180°C.

2. Line a baking tray or tin foil tray approx. 30 x 20 cm (12 x 8 inches) with non-stick baking paper.

3. Place the margarine, flour, sugar, syrup, treacle, vanilla extract/essence, eggs and cream into a bowl and mix with an electric mixer or wooden spoon until soft

4. Place the mixture in the baking tray and bake for 30-40 minutes until set

5. Leave to cool in the tin.

6. For the icing put the margarine, cream and brown sugar in a pan and stir all the time over a low heat until the margarine has melted and the sugar has dissolved. **Do not boil.**

7. Remove the pan from the heat and mix in the icing sugar.

8. Take the sponge out of the tin and drizzle the icing over the top and leave to set before cutting into equal sized pieces.

Oat Bars

Ingredients:

Porridge Oats • 150g
Sultanas • 200g
Wholemeal Self-Raising Flour • 100g
Granulated Sugar • 125g
Coconut • 50g
Butter or Margarine • 150g
Syrup • 2 level tablespoon

Serving Suggestions:

Dried cranberries, apricots, raisins or a mixture of dried fruit or chocolate chips/fudge pieces.

Method:

1. Set oven to Gas mark 4, 180°C.
2. Grease a baking tray or tin foil tray 30 x 20 cm approx (12 x 8 inches).
3. In a large bowl weigh the porridge oats, sultanas, flour, sugar and coconut.
4. Melt the butter/ margarine and sugar in a pan over a low heat (stirring with a woodenspoon). **Do not boil.**
5. Add this to the bowl of dry ingredients and mix well together using a wooden spoon or a fork if that's easier. The mixture should cling together.
6. Press the mixture evenly into the greased baking tray / tin foil tray and smooth the surface using the back of a clean tablespoon.
7. Bake for approx. 25 - 30 minutes (NB — the mixture will feel a little a soft at this stage).
8. Allow to cool slightly for about 10 minutes and then mark into pieces.
9. Leave in tray to cool completely before cutting right through into pieces.

Quick Banana Loaf

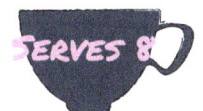
Serves 8

Ingredients:

Margarine · 75g
Caster Sugar · 150g
Eggs · 2 at room temperature (beaten)
Bananas (ripe) · 3 (mashed with a fork)
Plain Flour · 200g
Baking Powder · 3 level teaspoons
Salt · ½ level teaspoon

Method:

1. Set oven to Gas Mark 4, 180°C.
2. Lightly grease a 2lb loaf tin and place a piece of non-stick baking paper cut to size in the bottom (this makes it easier to turn out) or use a loaf tin liner.
3. Cream margarine and sugar.
4. Beat in eggs one at a time.
5. Beat in the mashed bananas and salt.
6. Stir in the flour and baking powder.
7. Turn into greased baking tin and bake for 60 -70 minutes until golden brown.
8. Bake for 35 minutes until golden brown and firm to touch (you could pierce it with a skewer or vegetable knife if wished and it should come out clean when it's ready).
9. Leave to cool for 5 minutes and then turn out of the tin.

Apple and Cranberry Cake

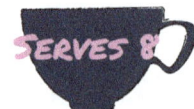

Serves 8

Ingredients:

Self-Raising Flour • 250g
Baking Powder • 5mls (1 teaspoon)
Caster Sugar • 200g
Eggs • 2 at room temperature
Almond Essence • 2.5ml (½ teaspoon)
Margarine or Butter (soft) • 150g
Eating Apples • 2 or 200g tinned apples
Dried Cranberries • 100g
Flaked Almonds • 25g (optional)

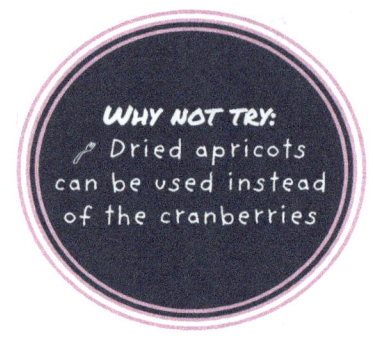

Why not try: Dried apricots can be used instead of the cranberries

Method:

1. Set oven to Gas mark 3, 170°C.

2. Grease a 20cm (8 inch) cake tin and line with a circle of non-stick baking paper in the bottom.

3. Wash the apples, cut into 4 and remove the core. Cut into thin slices OR cut up the tinned apples slightly.

4. Place the flour, baking powder, sugar, eggs, almond essence and margarine into a large baking bowl and beat with a wooden spoon or electric mixer until smooth.

5. Add the apples and cranberries to the cake mixture and gently mix.

6. Place the mixture into the lined cake tin and level the surface. Sprinkle the flaked almonds over the top if using.

7. Bake for 1 – 1½ hours until the cake is firm to the touch and golden brown.

8. Leave to cool in the tin for about 10 minutes and then turn out

Tiffin

Ingredients:

Margarine • 100g
Syrup • 2 tablespoons
Sultanas • 1 cup
Drinking Chocolate • 2 tablespoons
Rich Tea or Digestive Biscuits • 1 packet (300g)
Cooking Chocolate • 10 squares

Method:

1. Crush the biscuits in a food processor or in a plastic food bag with a rolling pin.
2. Place all the other ingredients into a pan and heat on a low heat until the margarine has melted. **Do not boil.**
3. Add the biscuits and mix well (add some extra biscuits if the mixture is too soft).
4. Place into a small round baking tin and smooth the surface with the back of a clean tablespoon. Set to one side to cool.
5. Melt the chocolate in a bowl over a pan of hot water or in the microwave.
6. Pour the melted chocolate over the top of the Tiffan and smooth with the back of a clean metal spoon.
7. Allow mixture to set before cutting (do not put it in the fridge as this will make hard to cut).

Why not try:
- Add some chocolate chips to the mixture before turning into the tin.
- You could sprinkle chocolate strands over the top of the melted chocolate.

Blueberry & White Chocolate Muffins

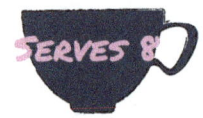

Ingredients:

Self-Raising Flour • 150g
Caster Sugar • 50g
Eggs • 1
Margarine • 50g
Milk • 100ml
Blueberries (fresh) • 75g
White Chocolate Pieces/Drops • 75g

Method:

1. Set oven to Gas Mark 5, 190°C.
2. Place 10 paper cake cases in a patty/bun tin.
3. Melt the margarine in a pan or in the microwave. **Do not boil.**
4. Place the flour and sugar into a baking bowl and mix.
5. Beat the egg in a jug and stir in the cooled melted margarine.
6. Add the contents of the jug to the dry ingredients and quickly mix in – don't over mix, it should still be lumpy. Add the chocolate pieces and blueberries and lightly mix in.
7. Spoon evenly into the paper cases (approximately 1 dessertspoon in each case).
8. Bake for about 15 minutes until well risen and golden brown.

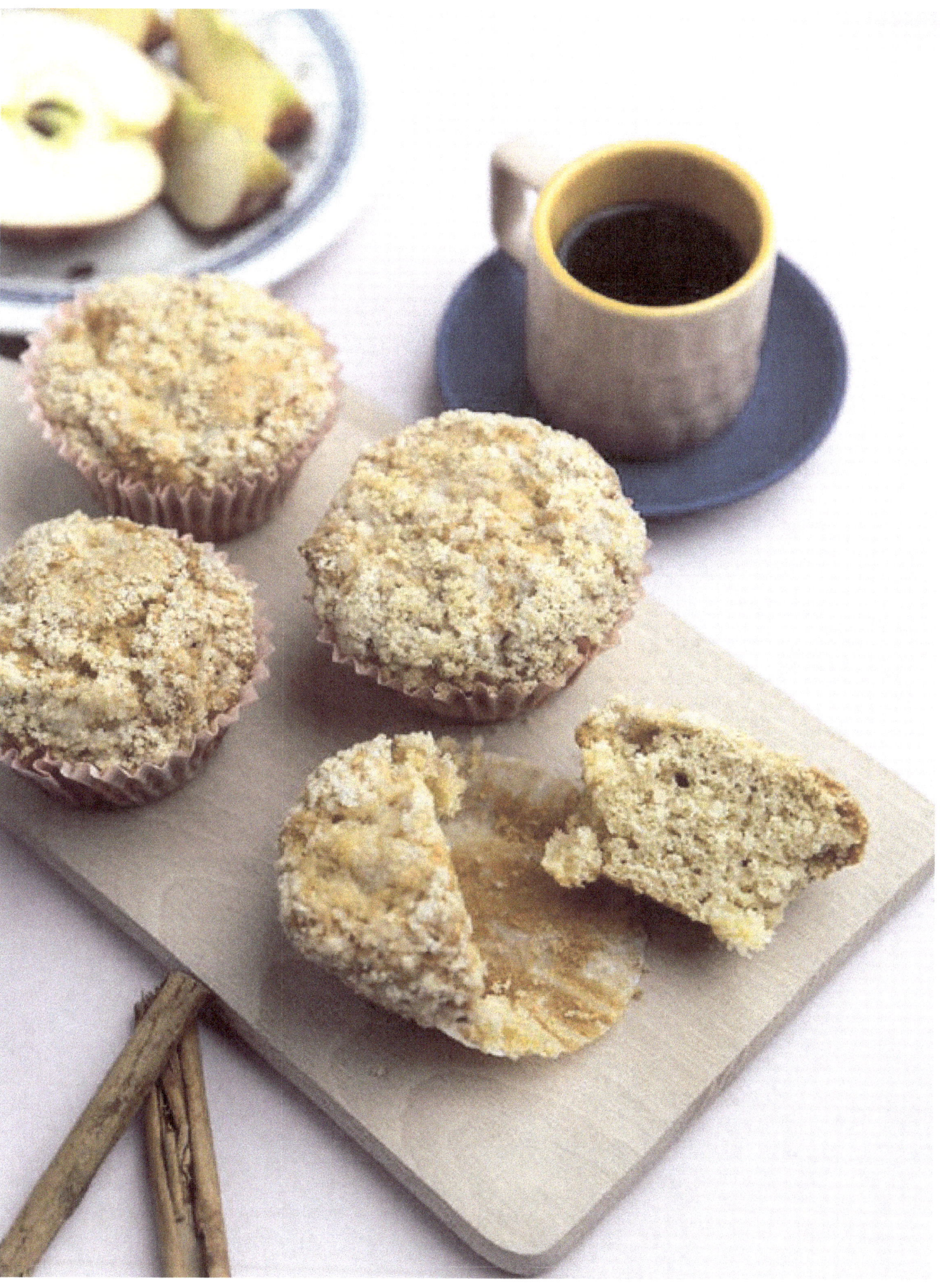

Warm Spiced Apple Pie Muffins

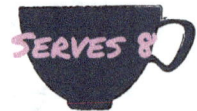
Serves 8

Ingredients:

Muffins:
Butter or Margarine (soft) • 50g
Demerara Sugar • 75g
Egg • 1 (lightly beaten)
Plain Flour • 150g
Baking Powder • 7.5mls (1½ teaspoons)
Mixed Spice (ground) • 2.5mls (½ teaspoon)
Cooking Apple • 1 large (peeled and chopped)
Fresh Orange Juice • 15mls (1 tablespoon)

Topping:
Plain Flour • 40g
Mixed Spice (ground) • 2.5mls (½ teaspoon)
Butter • 25g
Caster Sugar • 40g

Method:

1. Set oven to Gas Mark 4, 180°C.
2. Place 12 muffin cases in a muffin tin.

   Make topping:
3. Place all the ingredients for the topping in a bowl and rub in with the fingertips until the mixture resembles fine breadcrumbs and set to one side (this can be done in a food processor).

   Make muffins:
4. Place the butter and sugar in a large bowl and cream (beat together) until light and fluffy.
5. Gradually beat in the egg.
6. Sieve the flour, baking powder and mixed spice together then fold into the mixture.
7. Fold in the chopped apple and orange juice.
8. Divide the mixture between the muffin cases.
9. Cover the top of each of the muffins with the reserved topping mixture.
10. Bake for 30 minutes or until golden brown.
11. Leave muffins in the tin to cool slightly before transferring to a cooling tray.

Raspberry and Banana Muffins

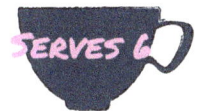
Serves 6

Ingredients:

Self-Raising Flour • 150g
Caster Sugar • 75g
Baking Powder • 5mls (1 teaspoon)
Margarine • 75g
Banana • 1 ripe
Eggs • 1 at room temperature (beaten)
Milk • 75ml
Fresh Raspberries • 75g
Soft Brown Sugar • 30ml for sprinkling on top
Sunflower or Pumpkin Seeds • 5ml (1 teaspoon) - optional

Method:

1. Set oven to Gas Mark 6, 200°C.
2. Place 6 muffin cases into a muffin tin.
3. Melt the margarine in a pan and leave to cool.
4. Peel and mash the banana. Break up the raspberries a little with a fork.
5. In a baking bowl place the flour, baking powder, caster sugar and stir to mix.
6. Add the milk and beaten egg into the margarine and mix together.
7. Add the milk mixture into the bowl with the flour mixture and mix together very lightly.
8. Add in the banana and raspberries but do not over mix — it will still look a bit lumpy
9. Divide the mixture between the cake cases and sprinkle a little brown sugar on top (and seeds if using)
10. Bake for 15 — 20 minutes until risen and firm.

Mango & Ginger Muffins

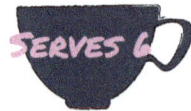
Serves 6

Ingredients:

Light Brown Sugar • 150g
Self-Raising Flour • 225g
Rolled Oats • 50g
Mixed Spice • 10mls (2 teaspoons)
Baking Powder • 5mls (1 teaspoon)
Dried Mango • 100g
Lazy Ginger • 2.5 ml
Eggs • 1 at room temperature
Vegetable Oil • 100ml
Milk • 175ml

Method:

1. Set oven to Gas Mark 6, 200°C.
2. Place 6 muffin cases into a muffin tin.
3. Cut up the dried mango into very small pieces.
4. Put the sugar, flour, oats, mango, ginger, mixed spice and baking powder into a bowl.
5. Mix the beaten egg, oil and milk together in a jug and add to the bowl of dry ingredients.
6. Beat the mixture together lightly with a wooden spoon until just mixed.
7. Divide the mixture equally between the paper cases and sprinkle a little extra oats on the top if wished.
8. Bake for 20 – 25 minutes until springy on the top and golden brown.
9. Cool in the tray for a couple of minutes then place onto a cooling tray

Why not try:

For a change place a small piece of pecan or almond on the top of each cake before cooking and after cooking drizzle a little glace icing over the top of each cake with a teaspoon (100g icing sugar and a little cold water – approx. 4-5 teaspoons – to mix)

Chocolate Muffins

Ingredients:

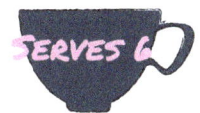 Serves 6

Plain Flour • 250mls
Baking Powder • 5mls (1 teaspoon)
Bicarbonate of Soda • 2.5mls (½ teaspoon)
Salt • Pinch
Cocoa Powder • 30mls
Drinking Chocolate • 30mls
Caster Sugar • 150g
Egg • 1
Milk • 250mls
Vegetable Oil • 90mls
Vanilla Essence • 5mls (1 teaspoon)

Method:

1. Set oven to Gas Mark 6, 200°C.
2. Place 6 muffin cases into a muffin tin.
3. Sieve flour, baking powder, bicarbonate of soda, salt, drinking chocolate and cocoa into a large bowl.
4. Stir sugar into bowl.
5. Measure oil and milk into a measuring jug.
6. Beat egg and vanilla in a cup.
7. Pour the contents from the measuring jug and cup into the bowl and stir until combined. The batter will be lumpy but no dry flour should be visible.
8. Pour cake batter into the measuring jug.
9. Fill the muffin cases ¾ full.
10. Bake for 20-25 minutes until tops spring back when touched.
11. Remove from muffin tins and cool on a cooling tray.

Flapjacks

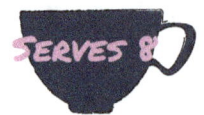
Serves 8

Ingredients:

Margarine • 50g
Soft Brown Sugar • 35g
Syrup • 10mls
Porridge Oats • 100g

Method:

1. Set oven to Gas Mark 5, 190°C.
2. Grease a small cake tin with a little soft margarine.
3. Place the margarine, syrup and sugar into a pan and heat on a low heat, stirring all the time until the mixture has melted (do not boil).
4. Stir in the Porridge Oats.
5. Place the mixture into the greased tin and smooth the surface with the back of a clean tablespoon.
6. Bake in the oven for 15 – 20 minutes until it springs back when touched.
7. Set to one side to cool.

Marshmallow Krispie Slice

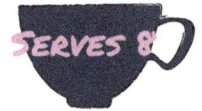
Serves 8

Ingredients:

Margarine • 100g
Toffee • 100g
Marshmallows • 100g
Rice Krispies • 125g

Method:

1. Place the margarine, toffee and marshmallows into a pan and heat on a low heat until the mixture has melted. **Do not boil.**
2. Add the Rice Krispies (add a little more if the mixture is too soft).
3. Place into a small round baking tin and smooth the surface with the back of a clean tablespoon. Set to one side to cool (do not put it in the fridge as this will make it too hard to cut).

Fudge Fingers

Ingredients:

Tinned Caramel • 1 tin
Biscuits such as Hob Nobs, Digestive, Ginger Nuts • 200g
Cooking Chocolate • 10 squares

Method:

1. Crush biscuits in either a food processor or polythene bag with a rolling pin (see Kitchen Journal).
2. Empty tin of caramel into a pan and warm through on a low heat, stirring all the time.
3. Remove from the heat and stir in the crushed biscuits.
4. Press mixture into a small sandwich tin.
5. Melt the chocolate in a bowl over a pan of hot water or in the microwave.
6. Pour the melted chocolate over the top of the biscuit mixture and smooth with the back of a clean metal spoon.
7. Allow mixture to set before cutting (do not put it in the fridge as this will make hard to cut).

Muesli Bars

Ingredients:

Good Quality Cooking Chocolate • 100g
Syrup • 3 x 15 ml
Margarine • 25g
Muesli • 225g

Method:

1. Melt the chocolate, syrup, and margarine in a pan over a low heat (stirring all the time) — It should only take about a minute or place in a bowl and microwave for about a minute until melted.
2. Add the muesli and mix well with a wooden spoon.
3. Place into a lightly greased round or square tin — about 20cm (8 inches).
4. Flatten with the back of a clean tablespoon.
5. Leave to firm and then cut into pieces.

No Bake Marshmallow Roll

Ingredients:

Marshmallows • 7
Digestive Biscuits (crushed) • 7
Condensed Milk • 2 tablespoons
Glace Cherries • 3
Coconut • 1 dessertspoon
Coconut for coating

Method:

1. Cut marshmallows into small pieces using scissors dipped in cold water.
2. Wash, dry, and cut up the cherries.
3. Place the cherries and marshmallows into a large bowl.
4. Add the crushed biscuits and dessertspoon of coconut to the bowl.
5. Add the condensed milk and bind the mixture together with a fork.
6. Place a piece of greaseproof paper on the work surface and sprinkle with a tablespoon of coconut.
7. Place the marshmallow mixture on to the greaseproof paper and roll into a sausage shape, coating it with the coconut.
8. Roll in the paper and place in the fridge until set (approximately 15-20 minutes)
9. Remove from the fridge once firm and cut into slices.

Belgian Loaf

Ingredients:

Caster Sugar • 1 cup
Milk • 1 cup
Sultanas • 1 cup
Margarine • 100g
Plain Flour • 2 cups
Baking Powder • ½ teaspoon
Baking Soda • ½ teaspoon
Eggs • 1 at room temperature (well beaten)

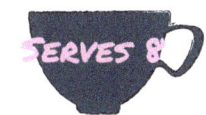

Method:

1. Set oven to Gas Mark 4, 180°C.

2. Lightly grease a 2lb loaf tin and place a piece of non-stick baking paper cut to size in the bottom (this makes it easier to turn out) or use a loaf tin liner.

3. Put the sugar, milk, sultanas, and margarine into a pan and bring slowly to the boil stirring all the time.

4. Stir in the flour, baking powder, baking soda and well beaten egg.

5. Turn into the greased loaf tin and bake for 60 minutes until golden brown and firm to touch (you could pierce it with a skewer or vegetable knife if wished and it should come out clean when it's ready).

6. Leave to cool for 5 minutes and then turn out of the tin.

Mix and Match Scones

Ingredients:

Basic Scone Recipe:
Self-Raising Flour · 250g
Baking Powder · 5mls
Salt · Pinch
Caster Sugar · 10mls (optional)
Margarine · 50g
Milk · 100mls (approx)

Method:

1. Set oven to Gas Mark 6, 200°C.
2. Lightly flour a baking tray.
3. Measure flour, baking powder and salt into a bowl.
4. Cut margarine into small pieces in bowl and rub in with flour until mixture resembles fine breadcrumbs. You can use a food processor to do this.
5. Add sugar and any fruit (if being used).
6. Mix with enough milk to make a soft, but not sticky dough.
7. Turn on to a floured tabletop, knead lightly and roll/flatten out to 2cm thickness.
8. Cut into rounds using a scone cutter or shape into a circle and cut into 8 wedges.
9. Place scones on to the floured baking tray leaving space between them.
10. Brush tops with a little milk or you can leave them floury topped.
11. Bake for 8-10 minutes or until golden brown.
12. Remove from oven and place on a cooling tray until cool.

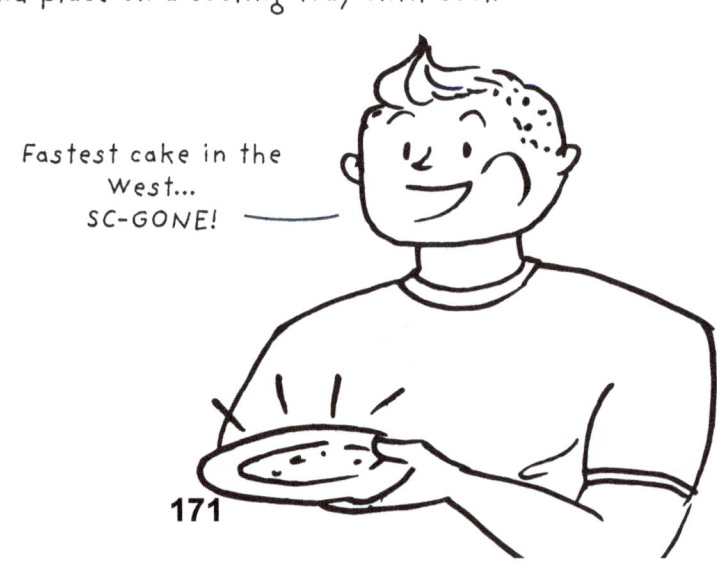

Fastest cake in the West... SC-GONE!

Mix and Match Scones

Choice of Flour:

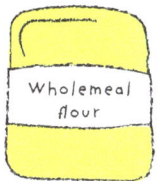 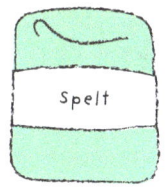 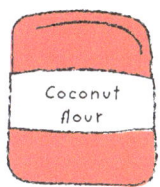 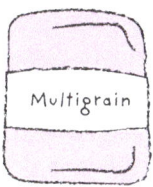 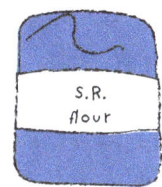

Choice of Fat:

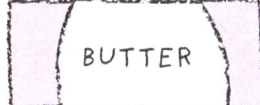 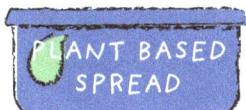 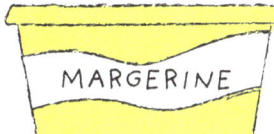 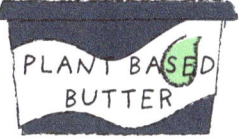

Choice of Fillings:

Strawberry pieces fresh or frozen · Raspberry pieces fresh or frozen
Black Cherry fresh or tinned (drained) · Blueberry fresh or frozen Fudge pieces
Sultanas / raisins · Chopped apricot · Chopped nuts / crushed Roasted Hazelnuts
Coconut · Lemon curd · Grated eating Apple · Grated Cheese (any type) ·
Cubes of Feta Cheese · Small pieces Cooked Ham/Bacon/Quorn ·
Small pieces Smoked Salmon · Chopped drained Sun-Dried Tomatoes
Chopped drained Jalepeno Peppers · Chopped drained Gherkins

Choice of Herbs:

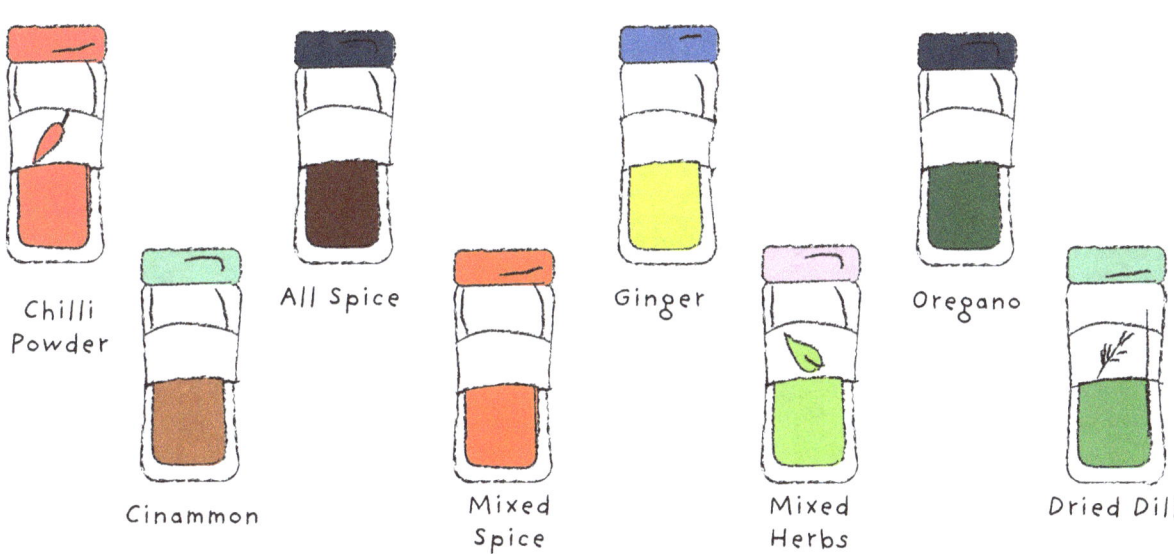

Choice of Glaze / Topping:

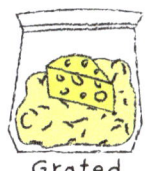 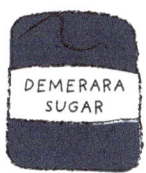 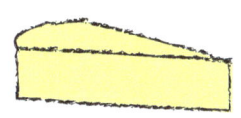 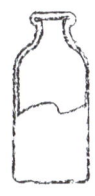 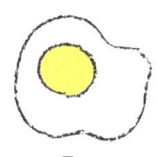

Grated Cheese · Demerara Sugar · Parmesan · Milk · Egg

Apple & Cinammon Scones

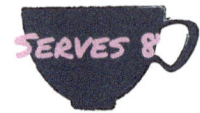
Serves 8

Ingredients:

Self-Raising Flour • 150g
Wholemeal Flour • 50g
Margarine • 50g
Baking Powder • 5mls
Cinnamon (ground) • 2.5mls
Caster Sugar • 5mls
Apple (eating) • 1 small
Milk to mix

Serving Suggestion:

Serve with softened butter and jam or some whipped or clotted cream and jam or fresh fruit.

Method:

1. Set oven to Gas Mark 6, 200°C.
2. Sieve the flours and baking powder into a large bowl.
3. Rub in margarine until mixture resembles fine breadcrumbs.
4. Grate the apple on to a plate (with skin on).
5. Add sugar, cinnamon and apple to the large bowl and stir to mix.
6. Using a knife stir in enough milk to make a soft, but not sticky dough.
7. Turn the mixture out on to a lightly floured table top and knead lightly until smooth.
8. Roll out until 2cm thick.
9. Cut into 6 or 8 even sized pieces.
10. Place on lightly floured baking tray.
11. Brush tops of scones with a little milk and sprinkle surface of milk with a little Demerara sugar.
12. Bake in a hot oven for 10-12 minutes or until golden brown and the bottom sounds hollow when tapped.
13. Transfer the scones to a cooling tray.

Cook's Tip

You can add sultanas to scones or change the apple for a pear.

Keep in an airtight container and use within 36 hours

Suitable for freezing (use within 3 months of freezing).

Sun-Dried Tomato & Cheese Scones

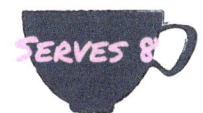
Serves 8

Ingredients:

Self-Raising Flour • 150g
Wholemeal Flour • 50g
Margarine • 50g
Baking Powder • 5mls
Sun-Dried Tomatoes (drained) • 25g
Cheese (grated or cubes) • 25g
Milk to mix

Serving Suggestion:

Serve with softened butter/herb butter or cream cheese and extra filling such as grated cheese / fresh tomato / cucumber.

Method:

1. Set oven to Gas Mark 6, 200°C.
2. Sieve the flours and baking powder into a large bowl.
3. Rub in margarine until mixture resembles fine breadcrumbs (this can be done in a food processor).
4. Drain and chop the Sun-dried Tomatoes and add to the bowl.
5. Add the cheese and stir to mix.
6. Using a knife stir in enough milk to make a soft, but not sticky dough.
7. Turn the mixture out on to a lightly floured table top and knead lightly until smooth.
8. Roll out until 2cm thick.
9. Cut into 6 or 8 even sized pieces.
10. Place on lightly floured baking tray.
11. Brush tops of scones with a little milk and sprinkle surface of milk with a little grated cheese (optional)
12. Bake in a hot oven for 10-12 minutes or until golden brown and the bottoms sound hollow when tapped.
13. Transfer the scones to a cooling tray.

RECIPE INDEX

Starters	Page Number
Cheesy Garlic Bread	16
Sun-Dried Tomato Rolls	17
Savoury Toasts	18
Chicken Filo Parcels	19
Turkey Meatballs with Cheese and Chive Dip	21
Tuna or Hot Smoked Salmon Pate with Toastie Soldiers	22
Fish Goujons with Tomato Salsa	23
Bruschetta	24
Tomato Salsa	25

Soups	Page Number
Tomato, Lentil and Red Pepper Soup	27
Cream of Lentil Soup with Croutons	28
Spicy Leek and Potato Soup	30
Butternut Squash and Sweet Potato Soup	31
Carrot and Sweet Potato Soup	32
Tomato and Bean Soup	33
Carrot and Courgette Soup	34
Tomato and Basil Soup	35
Mushroom, Sweet Potato, and Carrot Soup	36
Minestrone Soup	37
Lentil, Carrot and Apple Soup	39
Spicy Lentil Soup	40
Sweet Potato and Mixed Pepper Soup	41

Mains	Page Number
Chilli Con Carne	44
Cheesy Tuna Fishcakes	45
Smoked Haddock Risotto	46
Mix and Match Pizza	48
Mini Margarita Pizzas	50
Sweet Pizzas	51
Christmas Pizzas	52
Easter Bunny Pizza	53
Cheat's Lamb Curry	54
Cheat's Chicken Tikka	55
Spicy Chicken Risotto	56
Mozzarella and Chicken Bake	57
Spicy Meatballs with Cheese and Chive Dip	58
Chicken Pie	59
Mock Mousakka	60

Pizza Whirls	62
Vegetable Stir Fry	63
Moroccan Chicken	64
Couscous	65
Egg Fried Rice	67
Five-Spice Pork	68
Chicken Bake	69
Chicken, Chorizo and Butternut Squash Stew	70
Chicken Jamboree	71
Chicken and Mango Curry	72
Beef and Sweet Potato Casserole	73
Beef with Apricots	74
Cottage Pie with Sweet Potato Topping	75
Mediterranean Pork Casserole	76
Pork Medallions with Creamy Mustard Sauce	77
Sausage Stew	78
Mixed Bean Goulash	79
Fish Burgers with Tartare Sauce	80

Pasta	Page Number
Spaghetti Bolognaise	83
Macaroni Cheese	84
Chicken Supreme	85
Pasta Potage	86
Salmon Tagliatelle	87
Spicy Chicken Pasta	89
Minestrone Pasta Pot	90
Beef and Macaroni Bake	91
Arrabiata Pasta Sauce	92
All-in-one Mince and Pasta	93
Curried Beef and Tomato Pasta	94
Chorizo and Sweetcorn Bake	96
Pasta Carbonara	97

Desserts	Page Number
Strawberry Layer Cake	99
Chocolate Layer Cake	100
Vanilla Panna Cotta	101
Coriander, Lemongrass, and Pineapple Compote	102
Mandarin or Peach Gateau	104
Easy Fruity Yoghurt Dessert	105
Chilled Lemon Flan	106
Mixed Berry Shortcake	107
Sticky Toffee Pudding	109
Apple and Cinammon Parcels	110

Fruit Kebab with Chocolate Dip	111
White Chocolate and Lime Cheesecake	112
Lemon Posset with Honeycomb	114
Cheat's Tiramisu	115
Fruit Crumble Tart	116
Plate Apple Tart	117
Fruity Bread Pudding	118
Apple Crumble	119
Fruity Brioche Bread and Butter Pudding	120
Panettone Bread and Butter Pudding	121
Summer Fruit Brulee	122
Fruit Sponge Pudding	123
Strawberry and Almond Crumble	124
Chocolate Roulade	126
Apples Stuffed with Raspberries	127
Poached Pears with Chocolate Sauce	128
Mix and Match Cheesecake	129
Pecan, Maple, and Vanilla Cheesecake	131
White Chocolate and Jamaican Rum Cheesecake	132

Sweet Treats	**Page Number**
Crunch Biscuits	134
Oat and Sultana Cookies	135
Shortbread Biscuits	136
Dippy-Dunk Cookies	138
Valentine's Biscuits	139
Truffles	140
Malteser Slice	141
Bakewell Tart	142
Mix and Match Sponge Cakes	143
Monster Cakes	144
Individual Sponge Cakes	145
Butterfly Cake	146
Chocolate Butterfly Cakes	147
Jammy Layer Cake	148
Mini Apple Crumble Tarts	149
Mini Lemon Tarts	150
Bonfire Cake	151
Blueberry Crumble Traybake	153
Lemon Drizzle Cakes	154
Mars Bar Traybake	155
Sticky Toffee Traybake	156
Oat Bars	157
Quick Banana Loaf	158
Apple and Cranberry Cake	159
Tiffin	160

Pizza Whirls	62
Vegetable Stir Fry	63
Moroccan Chicken	64
Couscous	65
Egg Fried Rice	67
Five-Spice Pork	68
Chicken Bake	69
Chicken, Chorizo and Butternut Squash Stew	70
Chicken Jamboree	71
Chicken and Mango Curry	72
Beef and Sweet Potato Casserole	73
Beef with Apricots	74
Cottage Pie with Sweet Potato Topping	75
Mediterranean Pork Casserole	76
Pork Medallions with Creamy Mustard Sauce	77
Sausage Stew	78
Mixed Bean Goulash	79
Fish Burgers with Tartare Sauce	80

Pasta	Page Number
Spaghetti Bolognaise	83
Macaroni Cheese	84
Chicken Supreme	85
Pasta Potage	86
Salmon Tagliatelle	87
Spicy Chicken Pasta	89
Minestrone Pasta Pot	90
Beef and Macaroni Bake	91
Arrabiata Pasta Sauce	92
All-in-one Mince and Pasta	93
Curried Beef and Tomato Pasta	94
Chorizo and Sweetcorn Bake	96
Pasta Carbonara	97

Desserts	Page Number
Strawberry Layer Cake	99
Chocolate Layer Cake	100
Vanilla Panna Cotta	101
Coriander, Lemongrass, and Pineapple Compote	102
Mandarin or Peach Gateau	104
Easy Fruity Yoghurt Dessert	105
Chilled Lemon Flan	106
Mixed Berry Shortcake	107
Sticky Toffee Pudding	109
Apple and Cinammon Parcels	110

Fruit Kebab with Chocolate Dip	111
White Chocolate and Lime Cheesecake	112
Lemon Posset with Honeycomb	114
Cheat's Tiramisu	115
Fruit Crumble Tart	116
Plate Apple Tart	117
Fruity Bread Pudding	118
Apple Crumble	119
Fruity Brioche Bread and Butter Pudding	120
Panettone Bread and Butter Pudding	121
Summer Fruit Brulee	122
Fruit Sponge Pudding	123
Strawberry and Almond Crumble	124
Chocolate Roulade	126
Apples Stuffed with Raspberries	127
Poached Pears with Chocolate Sauce	128
Mix and Match Cheesecake	129
Pecan, Maple, and Vanilla Cheesecake	131
White Chocolate and Jamaican Rum Cheesecake	132

Sweet Treats	Page Number
Crunch Biscuits	134
Oat and Sultana Cookies	135
Shortbread Biscuits	136
Dippy-Dunk Cookies	138
Valentine's Biscuits	139
Truffles	140
Malteser Slice	141
Bakewell Tart	142
Mix and Match Sponge Cakes	143
Monster Cakes	144
Individual Sponge Cakes	145
Butterfly Cake	146
Chocolate Butterfly Cakes	147
Jammy Layer Cake	148
Mini Apple Crumble Tarts	149
Mini Lemon Tarts	150
Bonfire Cake	151
Blueberry Crumble Traybake	153
Lemon Drizzle Cakes	154
Mars Bar Traybake	155
Sticky Toffee Traybake	156
Oat Bars	157
Quick Banana Loaf	158
Apple and Cranberry Cake	159
Tiffin	160

Blueberry and White Chocolate Muffins	161
Warm Spiced Apple Pie Muffins	163
Raspberry and Banana Muffins	164
Mango and Ginger Muffins	165
Chocolate Muffins	166
Flapjacks	167
Marshmallow Krispie Slice	167
Fudge Fingers	168
Muesli Bars	168
No Bake Marshmallow Roll	169
Belgian Loaf	170
Mix and Match Scones	171
Apples and Cinammon Scones	173
Sun-Dried Tomato and Cheese Scones	174

www.ingramcontent.com/pod-product-compliance
Lightning Source LLC
Chambersburg PA
CBHW081617100526
44590CB00021B/3482